"*Introducing ASL-English Educational Interpreting* is exceptional in its practical insights, tackling the unspoken questions often faced in the field. Drs. Fitzmaurice and Cates skillfully weave together relatable experiences, compelling anecdotes, and real-world scenarios, making the book invaluable for both seasoned Educational Interpreters, interpreter educators, and those involved in Deaf education."

– **Jennifer Place-Lewis, MS, NIC:A,** *Project Director, South Caroline Educational Interpreting Center, Clemson University*

"This is the first comprehensive textbook for educational interpreters that explains in detail all of the complexities of interpreting within educational settings. Introducing ASL-English Educational Interpreting is a complete game changer that EVERY interpreter should read!"

– **M. Antwan Campbell, MPA, Ed:K-12,** *IDEA Consultant for Deaf and Hard of Hearing and, Interpreter Support, Office of Exceptional Children, North Carolina Department of Public Instruction*

"Dr. Fitzmaurice and Dr. Cates have completed what stakeholders in educational interpreting have needed for decades. They have acknowledged the profound impact that educational interpreters have on the overall academic, social, and emotional development of Deaf students. Introducing ASL-English Educational Interpreting provides the insights necessary for educational interpreters, administrators, and interpreter preparation program faculty to evaluate existing programs and consequently to effectively implement these best practices."

– **Julie Delkamiller, Ed.D., CI/CT,** *Associate Professor, Special Education and Communication Disorders, University of Nebraska at Omaha*

Introducing ASL-English Educational Interpreting

This textbook offers a clear and accessible introduction to educational interpreting, focusing on the unique demands of working with Deaf students in public school settings. Most interpreters begin their careers in these environments, often without specific preparation for the developmental and educational needs of Deaf children.

The book explores the structure of school interpreting, the roles of key stakeholders, and the language and literacy development of Deaf learners. It also examines interpreter responsibilities, practical strategies, and the day-to-day logistics of classroom work.

With guidance on interpreter assessment, tools for collaboration with teachers, and tips for creating inclusive classrooms, this is an essential resource for students in interpreting and related programs, as well as educators and practitioners seeking to support Deaf students more effectively.

Dr. Stephen Fitzmaurice is an Associate Professor of Interpreting: American Sign Language (ASL) and the lead faculty for the ASL-English Educational Interpreting program at Clemson University.

Dr. Deborah Cates is the Language Resources Coordinator at the Iowa School for the Deaf in the Outreach department. She oversees the administration of the Sign Language Proficiency Interview (SLPI) program, manages the Deaf language coaching program, supervises staff sign language interpreters, and provides professional development and support in the state of Iowa.

Translation Practices Explained

Series Editor: Christopher Mellinger

Translation Practices Explained is a series of coursebooks designed to help self-learners and students on translation and interpreting courses. Each volume focuses on a specific aspect of professional translation and interpreting practice, usually corresponding to courses available in translator- and interpreter-training institutions. The authors are practicing translators, interpreters, and/or translator or interpreter trainers. Although specialists, they explain their professional insights in a manner accessible to the wider learning public.

Each volume includes activities and exercises designed to help learners consolidate their knowledge, while updated reading lists and website addresses will also help individual learners gain further insight into the realities of professional practice.

Most recent titles in the series:

Translating for Museums, Galleries and Heritage Sites
Robert Neather

Patient-Centred Translation and Communication
Vicent Montalt-Resurrección, Isabel García-Izquierdo and Ana Muñoz-Miquel

Conference Interpreting Explained
Elisabet Tiselius

Translating Tourism
Stefania M. Maci and Cinzia G. Spinzi

Introducing ASL-English Educational Interpreting
Stephen Fitzmaurice and Deborah Cates

For more information on any of these and other titles, or to order, please go to www.routledge.com/Translation-Practices-Explained/book-series/TPE

Additional resources for Translation and Interpreting Studies are available on the Routledge Translation Studies Portal: http://routledgetranslationstudiesportal.com/

Introducing ASL-English Educational Interpreting

Stephen Fitzmaurice and Deborah Cates

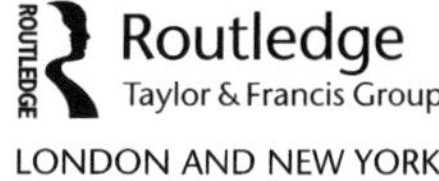

LONDON AND NEW YORK

Designed cover image: Getty Images. An open book. - stock illustration, @Ilya Lukichev

First published 2026
by Routledge
4 Park Square, Milton Park, Abingdon, Oxon OX14 4RN

and by Routledge
605 Third Avenue, New York, NY 10158

Routledge is an imprint of the Taylor & Francis Group, an informa business

Access the Student Resources: www.routledge.com/9781032729237

British Library Cataloguing-in-Publication Data
A catalogue record for this book is available from the British Library

Library of Congress Cataloging-in-Publication Data
A catalog record has been requested for this book

ISBN: 978-1-032-72921-3 (hbk)
ISBN: 978-1-032-72923-7 (pbk)
ISBN: 978-1-003-42305-8 (ebk)

DOI: 10.4324/9781003423058

Typeset in Sabon
by Taylor & Francis Books

Contents

Figures

Tables

Foreword

This volume, *Introducing ASL-English Educational Interpreting*, offers much more than a simple introduction to interpreting in educational settings. It provides deep insights into the varied contexts where interpreters not only interpret communication, but also act as professionals—supporting, advising, and contributing to the effective interactions and learning processes that educational systems are designed to foster.

I have spent many years researching, advocating for, and participating in the development of quality interpreting within educational environments. My journey began in the early 1980s when, as a student interpreter, I completed my first internship at a middle school. This was just a few years after the implementation of PL 94–142 (1975), a law aimed at providing free and appropriate education for children with disabilities in what were deemed the "least restrictive environments." While the intent was to integrate Deaf students into mainstream schools, these auditory-focused environments were not suited to their visual learning needs. The removal of Deaf children from residential schools, where their education centered around visual communication, often resulted in their isolation in public schools that were neither prepared nor equipped to meet their unique needs. As Dr. Oliva (2004) discusses in her work *Alone in the Mainstream*, this isolation has had long-term effects on the education of Deaf students. Although there has since been some research on the impacts of interpreted education, much of it remains underutilized or insufficiently implemented in real-world settings. Dr. Oliva notes that, despite advancements, little has changed for many Deaf students in these environments.

During the rollout of PL 94–142, passionate discussions emerged within the interpreting community about the practice of mainstreaming and educational interpreting. At the time, and even now, educational interpreters were often perceived as having unique challenges compared to their peers in other interpreting fields. Some even likened them to "mops expected to clean up the mess" caused by the law's implementation (Winston, 1990, p. 51). Rather than fostering improvement, the professional community frequently faced difficulties in offering training or support to those working in K-12 settings, further highlighting the opportunities for growth and development in educational environments.

My early experiences in this climate led to my first article, "Mainstreaming: Like it or Not" (Winston, 1985). In this piece, I made an appeal to the field to enhance, rather than hinder, the educational experiences of Deaf students. Since then, I have continued to research and advocate for better practices in the hope of improving these experiences.

Despite the many barriers that persist in the education of Deaf students, I was fortunate to begin my career in a setting where I worked alongside a dedicated teacher of the Deaf who prioritized the students' learning needs and championed strong communication, despite systemic limitations. Together, working as a team, we found creative ways to improve access, educate the school community, support Deaf students, and leverage our collective expertise to work as a team. It was through this experience that I began to explore the expectations, limitations, and successes of interpreted education.

Over the years, I have delved into questions of language access, interpreter ethics, and the visual needs of students in classrooms, to name a few. My first edited volume, *Educational Interpreting: How It Can Succeed* (Winston, 2004), was originally titled *Educational Interpreting: Why It Can't Succeed*, reflecting my frustration with the system's failures. However, at the editors' suggestion, I adopted a more hopeful and inviting title, recognizing that any progress made, even by a single individual who might read it, could improve the education of Deaf students. This volume was the first to address the needs of interpreters in education, supported by incorporating empirical research and emphasizing the contributions of such research to the field. While there have been advances in the preparation of educational interpreters, much work remains. This volume contributes to that ongoing dialogue by addressing areas in need of further understanding and research by educational systems and interpreters alike.

In my exploration of interpreted education, I have been privileged to work with many dedicated professionals. Two of them, Dr. Stephen Fitzmaurice and Dr. Deborah Cates, are the authors of this text. I first collaborated with Dr. Cates on another edited volume, where her chapter, "The Impact of Sign Language Interpreter Skill on Education Outcomes in K–12 Settings" (Cates & Delkamiller, 2021), demonstrated the significant effect interpreter qualifications have on the success of Deaf students. These findings remain crucial for educators, parents, and interpreters, underscoring the need for skilled professionals in these roles.

I have also worked closely with Dr. Fitzmaurice in various capacities over the years, from faculty collaborations to co-editing projects. His research, particularly his volume based on his dissertation on *The Role of the Educational Interpreter* (Fitzmaurice, 2021), has helped shift the perception of interpreters from passive facilitators to active partners within the educational system. His work encourages interpreters to take a more integrated role in supporting the Individualized Education Program (IEP) team and the broader educational process.

Introducing ASL-English Educational Interpreting provides all stakeholders—interpreters, educators, parents, and support personnel—with the tools to understand the far-reaching impacts of interpreted education. The authors begin by tracing the history of Deaf education and the challenges it has faced, highlighting the differences between interpreting for adults and for Deaf children who are still acquiring sign language. They then explore the broader educational systems where interpreting takes place, offering crucial insights into how interpreters can integrate their work into these settings.

The authors also delve into the complex relationships between the many individuals involved in a student's education, from teachers to administrators to audiologists, all people with whom interpreters must collaborate to ensure successful outcomes. This is followed up by an in-depth focus on the students themselves, examining the diverse experiences of Deaf, hard of hearing, and Deaf-Blind students, and the challenges they face both academically and socially.

The preceding discussions build up to the final chapter, where the authors narrow their focus to the specific role of interpreters in educational settings, emphasizing that they must first and foremost be highly qualified professionals. Beyond facilitating communication, they must align their work with the goals of the IEP and collaborate with the educational team to support the student's learning.

Each chapter of *Introducing ASL-English Educational Interpreting* offers valuable insights that can significantly improve the educational experiences of Deaf students. Taken as a whole, this volume serves as a comprehensive textbook for those looking to enter the field of educational interpreting, as well as an invaluable support for every person involved in educating Deaf students. The authors, drawing on their extensive knowledge and experience, have crafted a resource that will benefit anyone seeking to better understand the complexities of interpreting in educational settings. It is my hope that this text will continue to contribute to the ongoing progress in this field, helping to ensure that Deaf students receive the education they deserve.

Acknowledgements

This text would not be possible without the lessons we have learned from the Deaf students and adults we have worked with over the years. Naturally, we cannot name them all, but we thank you each for teaching and continuing to teach us. We also want to acknowledge our working educational interpreters. Your diligence in the work you do every day benefits Deaf students, Deaf communities, and the education system as a whole. We have learned much from our own experiences as educational interpreters and our continued work with current educational interpreters.

We also want to profoundly thank Dr. Betsy Winston for her gracious Foreword. Dr. Winston is a formidable researcher, author, and teacher, with experience in this field spanning 40 years. Interpreting communities have reaped many benefits from her diligent work, and Stephen has been fortunate to know Dr. Winston personally since 2005. She constantly asks the truly difficult questions of the system and us, challenging us to do better and be better for Deaf students. Stephen notes he is a better professional interpreter and educator because of Dr. Winston. Her research on discourse has also had a profound impact on Deborah's teaching approach. Dr. Winston's aspiration and inspiration are contagious.

To Deborah's colleagues at the Iowa School for the Deaf, especially Tina Caloud and John Cool, who have supported and promoted her work with educational interpreters, she would not be here without you. And, Jennifer Place-Lewis' commitment to reading and rereading drafts of what you are about to embark on, and her patience with helping us address our own blind spots and bad writing, are forever appreciated. Deborah's educational interpreter colleagues, Mary Mowry, Janay Eckrich, Kristina Dalen, and Nancy Pietrzak, graciously read early drafts of her chapters and provided their perspectives as current practitioners in the field. We also thank Dr. Chris Mellinger for his diligent and insightful editing suggestions.

Lastly, to our families. It is no small task to write a textbook, and our families have sacrificed their time with us so that we can bring this text to you. Deborah would especially like to thank her husband Blake, whose dedication to promoting her work–life balance has kept her sane.

List of Acronyms and Abbreviations

To ease your reading as you move through this text, we offer the following definitions for many of the acronyms we tend to use. There is a complete glossary for other acronyms and abbreviations at the end.

American Sign Language (ASL): a natural language with complete and organized features used by Deaf communities in the United States and Canada.

Americans with Disabilities Act (ADA): United States federal Public Law 101–336 which prohibits private sector employers and all state and local governments from discriminating against individuals with disabilities.

Contact Sign: a communication system that arises from contact with Deaf people using ASL and those using some form of Manually Coded English (MCE). Formerly known as Pidgin Signed English (PSE).

Free and Appropriate Public Education (FAPE): a legal right guaranteed under the Individuals with Disabilities Education Act (IDEA) or PL 94–142 in the United States. A FAPE ensures that students with disabilities receive special education and related services at no cost to the parents, is designed to meet their individual needs, and designed to help them make meaningful educational progress.

Individualized Education Program (IEP): a legal document detailing how a student with a disability is to receive a Free Appropriate Public Education (FAPE) in the United States. The IEP has identified team members and is jointly developed by members of the IEP Team and the student's parents.

Individuals with Disabilities Education Act (IDEA): United States federal Public Law 94–142, which ensures students with disabilities are provided with a Free Appropriate Public Education (FAPE). Formally this 1975 law was named the Education for All Handicapped Children Act.

Manually Coded English (MCE): an umbrella term for several sign systems that were invented in an attempt to visually represent the morphology and syntax of English using signs, fingerspelling, and invented markers. Unlike natural signed languages (like ASL), MCE is not a natural language, but an artificial system designed to show spoken or written English word-for-word in visual form and it is not predominantly used by Deaf communities.

Office of Special Education Services (OSES): a division at the federal and state Department of Education responsible for overseeing and ensuring compliance with federal and state regulations related to special education in the United

States. The OSES supports school districts in implementing the Individuals with Disabilities Education Act (IDEA) by providing guidance, resources, monitoring, and technical assistance to ensure that students with disabilities receive a Free Appropriate Public Education (FAPE) in the Least Restrictive Environment (LRE). Some school districts also call their special education division the Office of Special Education Services and these divisions are typically headed by the Director of Special Education.

References

Cates, D., & Delkamiller, J. (2021). The impact of sign language interpreter skill on education outcomes in K–12 settings. In E. Winston & S. B. Fitzmaurice (Eds.), *Advances in educational interpreting* (pp. 19–30). Washington, DC: Gallaudet University Press.

Fitzmaurice, S. B. (2021). *The role of the educational interpreter: Perceptions of administrators and teachers*. Washington, DC: Gallaudet University Press.

Oliva, G. (2004). *Alone in the mainstream: A deaf woman remembers public school*. Washington, DC: Gallaudet University Press.

Winston, E. A. (1985). Mainstreaming: Like it or not. *Journal of Interpretation*, 2, 117–119.

Winston, E. A. (1990). Mainstream interpreting: An analysis of the task. In L. Swabey (Ed.), *Proceedings of the eighth national convention of the Conference of Interpreter Trainers* (pp. 51–67). Pomona, CA: CIT Publications.

Winston, E. A. (2004). *Educational interpreting: How it can succeed*. Washington, DC: Gallaudet University Press.

1 Preface

We offer *Introducing ASL-English Educational Interpreting* as a primer for what the work of an educational sign language interpreter involves (hereafter educational interpreter). This text focuses specifically on ASL-English interpreting for Deaf students in educational settings in the United States. Many sign language interpreter programs have individual courses on educational interpreting and many two-year interpreter programs are a direct feed to the educational interpreting field. Having been educational interpreters, there are many things we wished we knew before we started. Our extensive experience working as and with educational interpreters allows us to easily recognize what interpreting curricula might need to address in order to prepare the next generation of educational interpreters.

We also know most of you are reading this text as you are studying the ASL-English interpreting field. For that reason, we do not delve deeply into the reader's cultural knowledge of Deaf peoples, Deaf history, art, literature, values, or other content areas about the Deaf experience. We also do not address the linguistics of American Sign Language (ASL), the general development of interpreting skills, nor general interpreting knowledge.

If you are a spoken language interpreter working in educational settings, much of this text may be of benefit to you. We also highly recommend you seek out other resources such as Kibbee (2016) for insight into how language intersects with legal rights and social equity. We also recommend reading Mellinger's (2021) examination on how spoken language interpreters work among students, families, and educational institutions. Mellinger highlights a number of unique spoken language interpreter challenges including policies and a complex educational environment.

There is ample research on the complex and multifaceted field of ASL-English educational interpreting. This research often focuses on interpreter role and duties, how much information an educational interpreter is conveying, or the current flawed system of practice. Most of this research is found in a multitude of research articles and texts which we will cite throughout.

Although this research is of tremendous value to academics, often these publications are not easily read by undergraduate students and do not adequately detail the knowledges, skills, and abilities that educational interpreters need to know before starting their work. In addition, as part of our experience

DOI: 10.4324/9781003423058-1

teaching educational interpreting to undergraduate students, we find most of the information on educational interpreting to be disparate, making us cobble together resources from all over the place rather than being able to rely on a compendium to support student learning.

Johnson, Taylor, Schick, Brown, and Bolster (2018) state in their first edition findings that "systemic change is desperately needed" (p. viii). They identify gaps in educational interpreter preparation in terms of both knowledge and skill, gaps in state-level and federal-level protections for Deaf student rights in education, and gaps in appropriate oversight of working educational interpreters. We cannot agree more, and this text is the result of our effort to better equip interpreting educators and students as we prepare educational interpreters before they enter the field.

Our Perspectives

Deaf Gain

Deaf Gain is the opposite of a deficit model of deafness. Rather than focusing on "hearing loss," Deaf Gain focuses on the benefits that Deaf people and signed languages have contributed to society, as well as personal benefits of being Deaf. For example, the huddle that is used in football was developed for Deaf football players at Gallaudet University. Another example is cross-cultural in that when Deaf people meet other Deaf people from around the world who use a different signed language, they have an easier time communicating than hearing people meeting speakers of other languages because the manual modality allows for more iconicity than the spoken modality, thus promoting more complex cross-cultural gestural communication (Whynot, 2016).

We believe that a fundamental shift is needed in Deaf Education so that the focus is on Deaf Gain (Alfrey & Jeanes, 2023; Bauman & Murray, 2009; 2014; Sheneman & Robinson, 2021; Skutnabb-Kangas, 2014). We believe that a deficit model of deafness is harmful to the educational outcomes of Deaf children. We believe that approaches to Deaf Education that emphasize audiological status rob Deaf children of language, identity, social emotional well-being, and education, often through the vehicle of language deprivation. Furthermore, such approaches relegate ASL to a "mode of communication," a tool to be used to supplement English, rather than recognizing it as a language in its own right.

Language Deprivation

We believe that the greatest threat to a Deaf child's education is the lack of accessible language early in life, referred to as *language deprivation* or *language delay*. Language deprivation carries the connotation of something being done *to* the child, whereas *language delay* carries the connotation of something being wrong *within* the child. We use the term language deprivation in this text as we believe that decisions made by adults and professionals in the child's life deprive the child of accessible language from birth. The resulting language delays that the child has are more often than not due to language deprivation rather than some inherent specific language disorder. As a result of language deprivation, many Deaf children start their formal education without a complete first language. Therefore, educational interpreters are tasked with supporting the child's first language development while also attempting to interpret. We address language deprivation and its impact on educational interpreters and Deaf students in detail in chapter six on language and literacy.

Use of "Big-D Deaf"

Once a child needs to access the classroom through visual language or with visual language support, we adopt the social definition of Deaf. Generally, in many texts, "D" (Big-D) Deaf means a cultural definition of deafness whereas "d" (Little-D) deaf indicates a level of hearing loss or an audiological focus (Padden & Humphries, 1988). We do not view Deaf children through a "what can you hear, what can't you hear" lens while engaging in educational interpreting. Therefore, we are not digressing from that norm by acknowledging the cultural aspects within Deaf communities.

We also recognize not all Deaf students have encultured or will enculture as a Deaf person. We recognize that Deaf students may self-identify as deaf, Deaf, hard-of-hearing, DeafBlind, DeafAnd, DeafPlus, DeafDisabled, Black Deaf, Indigenous Deaf, and many other multifaceted and intersectional identities. We absolutely respect and support every student's right to their own identity. However, we note that the emphasis on "deaf or hard of hearing" in the educational realm, really, is audiological in focus and perpetuates audism (see chapter four). In other words, throughout this text, we use Deaf to include all students who use visual language to access their school community.

Conveying ASL and Fingerspelling in Print

For ease of use we also generally use small caps to convey a word or morpheme that is produced in ASL. For example, TREE indicates that that item is signed. If an item is fingerspelled, we separate each letter with hyphens such as: W-I-L-L-I-A-M.

How We Talk about Interpreting Work

We note that some literature talks about the ASL-English interpreting process using phrases such as "interpreting from sign to voice" or "working from voice to sign" or "voicing for a Deaf person." This terminology confounds language and modality, which is a significant issue in the field of educational interpreting (see chapter three) (Fitzmaurice, 2024). To mitigate this, we rely heavily on our spoken language counterparts. Interpreters working between two languages reference both of those languages in discussing their work, using phrases such as "the interpreter was working from English to Spanish," or "I was interpreting from French to Japanese," etc. For our purposes, we use the same conventions and identify the source and target languages (i.e., "ASL-English" interpreters).

If you think about it, using "voice" makes no sense; a voice is a tool produced by the larynx, mouth, and vocal cords. It also represents agency, as in "having a voice" or "offering a dissenting voice." If you see voice as a tool, fingers would be an equivalent tool. Thus "fingers to voice" or "interpreting from voice to fingers." Again, it does not make sense. In any case, the use of "voice" and "sign" puts an emphasis on the modality, not on the language.

Similarly, the use of the phrase "ASL interpreter" completely ignores the English-speaking participants in the conversation. This also places emphasis on the Deaf person—who often is not the one who needs the interpreter! It may come as a surprise, but it is hearing people who need the interpreter to make their information accessible. The use of "ASL interpreter" implies that we only interpret into ASL, which further implies that our work is unidirectional—that we are there to give the Deaf person access to the hearing person but not vice versa. Terminology and labeling have a powerful effect on how we think about a thing, so using "ASL-English interpreter" promotes a framing of ASL as a language, the work of interpreting as a two-way street, and ASL and English as equally important languages for the work we do.

Use of "PSE"

We also know that not all students will use ASL, but they may well use a variety of Contact Sign. Historically, Contact Sign has wrongly been referred to as Pidgin Signed English or PSE. This is a linguistic misnomer (Lucas & Valli, 1989; Monikowski, 2004; Valli, Lucas, & Mulrooney, 2011). A pidgin is a simplified form of language used as a temporary measure between people not sharing a common language. Pidgins are constructed impromptu and are generally unsophisticated borrowing from elements of both languages (Lucas & Valli, 1989; Monikowski, 2004; Valli, Lucas, & Mulrooney, 2011). As such, it is impossible to have a pidgin with languages of a different modality. For example, you cannot use ASL and English in the same sentence, such as (English in italics, ASL in caps): *Hi, my*NAME*is*S-T-E-P-H-E-N*how are* YOU? In English all that is said is: Hi, my, is, how, are. And in ASL: NAME, S-T-E-P-H-E-N, YOU. Neither party has access to the entire pidgin message. Complicated? Yes. For our purposes, we know PSE is not a temporary feature—it has been around for many years and is absolutely the wrong terminology (we discuss this in more detail in chapter six). We use the more accurate term "Contact Sign" to indicate contact between Manual Codes of English (MCE) and ASL (Valli, Lucas, & Mulrooney, 2011).

How This Text is Structured

Introducing ASL-English Educational Interpreting is focused on the work of educational interpreters, or interpreters working in PK-12 education settings, and the added specialized competencies required for those settings. That is not to say interpreting in colleges and universities is not within an educational environment, simply that interpreting in colleges looks more similar to community-based interpreting (however, much of what we include herein is also applicable in those other environments).

This text is broadly separated into ten chapters, the first chapter being this preface. Chapter two, the "Introduction," details how interpreting in educational settings involves unique developmental, legal, and situational complexities, particularly when working with Deaf children who may experience language deprivation. Educational interpreters are legally recognized as Related Service Providers under the Individuals with Disabilities Education Act (IDEA), requiring them to support Individualized Education Program (IEP) goals and to collaborate closely with school staff. This volume highlights the evolving challenges of interpreted education and calls for better practices and professional recognition for interpreters in mainstream and Deaf education contexts.

"The System, Constituents, and Stakeholders," chapter three, examines how the US education system serves Deaf students, emphasizing the legal foundations of special education and the interpreter's role in supporting IEP goals under IDEA. It contrasts deficit-focused special education models with Deaf Education's focus on language access and cultural identity, highlighting tensions in placement decisions. The chapter underscores interpreters' expanded responsibilities, legal and ethical obligations, and the need for culturally affirming, linguistically accessible education shaped by Deaf perspectives.

From there, chapter four, "The Curriculum and Academic Content Areas," emphasizes the importance of academic standards and curriculum in shaping both classroom instruction and interpreter decision-making. It highlights the need for educational interpreters to possess broad extralinguistic knowledge, especially when interpreting assessments and subject-specific content. Additionally, it addresses interpreter roles beyond the classroom, including field trips, assemblies, and extracurricular activities.

Chapter five, "Deaf Students," explores the multifaceted role of educational interpreters in supporting Deaf students, emphasizing cultural competence, intersectionality, and systemic advocacy. It highlights the importance of recognizing Deafness as a cultural identity, understanding the unique needs of marginalized Deaf students, and using appropriate services such as Deaf Interpreters or Language Coaches to promote Deaf student language acquisition. The chapter also underscores the critical balance between assistive technology use and human interpretation, advocating for professional development and systemic change to ensure equitable, language-rich access to education.

"Language and Literacy," chapter six, highlights the importance of early access to a natural language like ASL in Deaf education, emphasizing its foundational role in cognitive, social, and academic development. It examines the negative impacts of language deprivation, critiques artificial sign systems for lacking sufficient linguistic depth, and outlines the unique literacy challenges Deaf students face using the Simple View of Reading. The chapter underscores the educational interpreter's critical role in supporting vocabulary development and creating language-rich environments that promote cognitive and academic growth.

The evolving role of educational interpreters is the focus of chapter seven, "Interpreting Processes and Decision-Making." By analyzing ethical frameworks, interpreting models, and role metaphors, this chapter also reintroduces the Partners in Education (PIE) metaphor to more accurately reflect the educational interpreter's dynamic responsibilities, including advocacy, instructional support, and collaboration within educational teams. The chapter emphasizes the importance of ethical flexibility, cultural humility, and practical decision-making models to guide interpreters in meeting the diverse and complex needs of Deaf students in educational settings.

Chapter eight, the final major chapter, "Logistics of Educational Interpreting," describes in depth the ways in which educational interpreting is a cognitively and emotionally demanding profession that requires both mental agility and key personality traits like empathy, flexibility, and emotional stability to navigate complex linguistic tasks and systemic challenges. Interpreters must balance advocacy, instruction, and ethical decision-making, often with minimal supervision, while tools like the Educational Interpreter Performance Assessment (EIPA) assess performance but fall short of national certification. The chapter highlights the importance of extralinguistic knowledge, preparation, and self-care strategies to manage stress, prevent burnout, and support Deaf students' access and autonomy in diverse educational settings.

Beyond that, we share our final thoughts in chapter nine and provide a general glossary. Each chapter includes thought questions based on the chapter information and a brief chapter summary.

References

Alfrey, L., & Jeanes, R. (2023). Challenging ableism and the 'disability as problem' discourse: How initial teacher education can support the inclusion of students with a disability in physical education. *Sport, Education and Society*, 28(3), 286–299.

Bauman, H. D., & Murray, J. (2009). Reframing: From hearing loss to deaf gain. *Deaf Studies Digital Journal*, 1(1), 1–10. https://www.researchgate.net/profile/Dirksen-Bauman-2/publication/264845480_Reframing_From_Hearing_Loss_to_Deaf_Gain/links/5d1c0279a6fdcc2462bacfd1/Reframing-From-Hearing-Loss-to-Deaf-Gain.pdf.

Bauman, H-D. L., & Murray, J. J. (Eds.) (2014). *Deaf gain: Raising the stakes for human diversity*. Minneapolis: University of Minnesota Press.

Fitzmaurice, S. (2024). Food for thought: Terms matter. *VIEWS*, 41(4), 24–25.

Johnson, L., Taylor, M., Schick, B., Brown, S., & Bolster, L. (2018). *Complexities in educational interpreting: An investigation into patterns of practice*. Edmonton: Interpreting Consolidated.

Kibbee, D. A. (2016). *Language and the law: Linguistic inequality in America*. Cambridge: Cambridge University Press.

Lucas, C., & Valli, C. (1989). Language contact in the American deaf community. In C. Lucas (Ed.), *The sociolinguistics of the Deaf community* (pp. 11–40). Cambridge, MA: Academic Press.

Mellinger, C. D. (2021). Interpreting and language access: Spoken Language Interpreters in U.S. educational contexts. In E. A. Winston & S. B. Fitzmaurice (Eds.), *Advances in Educational Interpreting* (pp. 44–67). Washington, DC: Gallaudet University Press.

Monikowski, C. (2004). Language myths in interpreted education: First language, second language, what language? In E. A. Winston (Ed.), *Educational interpreting: How it can succeed* (pp. 48–60). Washington, DC: Gallaudet University Press.

Padden, C., & Humphries, T. (1988). *Deaf in America: Voices from a culture.* Cambridge, MA: Harvard University Press.

Sheneman, N., & Robinson, O. E. (2021). Helpers, professional authority, and pathologized bodies: Ableism in interpretation and translation. In O. Carbonell i Cortés & E. Monzó-Nebot (Eds.), *Translating asymmetry–Rewriting power* (pp. 55–75). Amsterdam: John Benjamins.

Skutnabb-Kangas, T. (2014). Afterword. Implications of deaf gain: Linguistic human rights for deaf citizens. In H-D. L. Bauman & J. J. Murray (Eds.), *Deaf gain: Raising the stakes for human diversity* (pp. 492–502). Minneapolis: University of Minnesota Press.

Valli, C., Lucas, C., & Mulrooney, K. (2011). *Linguistics of American Sign Language: An introduction* (5th ed.). Washington, DC: Gallaudet University Press.

Whynot, L. (2016). *Understanding International Sign: A sociolinguistic study.* Washington, DC: Gallaudet University Press.

2 Introduction

Interpreter preparation programs primarily use materials and curricula designed to teach interpreters to work with adults who have a fully functional language. However, educational interpreting is fundamentally different. This chapter explores how developmental, legal, and situational considerations shape the role of educational interpreters, and advocates for recognizing educational interpreters as essential educational professionals supporting equitable access for Deaf students.

Developmental Considerations

Humans acquire social language and are taught academic language in childhood. Social language is acquired at home, and academic language is typically learned through formal education. Deaf children in mainstream settings usually have the distinct disadvantage of limited access to fluent adult and peer language models, both at school and at home.

Furthermore, due to the prevalence of language deprivation among Deaf children, many begin their formal education without a sufficient linguistic repertoire in either American Sign Language (ASL), as a first language, or English (B. Cerney, 2007; Cheng, Roth, Halgren, & Mayberry, 2019; Friedmann & Rusou, 2015; Hall, 2017; Hall, Hall, & Caselli, 2019). Therefore, educational interpreters are, by default, providing language modeling and direct instruction during the time when they are supposed to be interpreting academic content instruction (Fitzmaurice, 2017; 2021b; 2021c; Lawson, 2021). General education classrooms afford neither the time nor the stimuli required to do both language modeling and interpreting, so one must always be sacrificed for the other.

During their primary schooling, Deaf children are also learning how to use interpreters. Very young children are not able to distinguish interpreters from teachers, paraeducators, or other adults in the environment. In general, they do not understand that what the interpreter is saying is generally not coming from the interpreter themselves but from the teacher. Deaf students often cannot separate how well they understand their interpreter from how well they understand the content. If the interpreter is not structuring their interpretation in a way that the Deaf student *can* understand, the Deaf student likely does not

DOI: 10.4324/9781003423058-2

know that the interpretation and not their own comprehension is at fault. Therefore, educational interpreters must be linguistically flexible enough to interpret information in different ways, and should seek external evaluations of and feedback on their interpreting work.

Legal Considerations

Educational settings are governed by several laws in the United States that will be discussed in this text. Many countries around the globe have similar laws, so if you work in another country, refer to those specific laws. For example, in the United Kingdom, Deaf students fall under the Children and Families Act (United Kingdom Government, 2014) and the Special Educational Needs and Disability (SEND) Code of Practice: 0 to 25 years (Department for Education & Department of Health, 2015). In Canada, there is the Canadian Charter of Rights and Freedoms (Government of Canada, 1982) and many statutes fall under the provincial codes (Government of British Columbia, 1996; Government of Ontario, 1990). South Africa uses the South African Schools Act and several white papers (Department of Education, 2001; Republic of South Africa, 1996). Again, this text is written for ASL-English educational interpreting in the United States.

Educational interpreters have a legal designation as Related Service Providers who provide language and cultural access in both ASL and English to support Deaf students in benefitting from their educational programming. This means that educational interpreters are part of the Individualized Education Program (IEP) team. Educational interpreters' decisions must always be guided by the IEP, a consideration that does not exist in general community interpreting settings. The IEP is a legal document, and IEP violations carry significant consequences.

Although all interpreters are ethically bound by confidentiality, the way this plays out in educational settings is unique. Educational interpreters are members of the IEP Team, and as such bring language- and access-related concerns and recommendations to the IEP Team. However, sharing information outside of the IEP Team is more than just a violation of an ethical tenet—it is illegal under the Family Educational Rights and Privacy Act (FERPA). Furthermore, educational interpreters are often considered mandated reporters under child protection laws, meaning they are legally obligated to report any suspected abuse, neglect, or other threats to a child's well-being (Child Welfare Information Gateway, 2023). This obligation overrides professional confidentiality when the safety of a child is at risk. It is important to note that interpreter confidentiality—maintaining privacy in professional interactions—is not the same as privileged communication, which applies to specific professions such as lawyers, clergy, or therapists. Unlike those roles, educational interpreters do not have a legal privilege that exempts them from disclosing concerns about abuse or harm.

As mandated reporters, interpreters must report any reasonable suspicion of endangerment, including physical, emotional, or sexual abuse, neglect, or exposure to dangerous situations. They are not required to confirm abuse, only to report concerns to the appropriate authorities, such as a designated school official or child protection agency. Additionally, educational interpreters are responsible for reporting observed violations of the school's code of conduct, especially if such behavior poses risks to the safety or integrity of the educational environment.

Situational Considerations

Educational interpreters work in schools. There are certain expectations of any adult working in an educational environment. While some educational interpreters work part-time, the vast majority are full-time employees or contracted providers of a school district. As a school staff member, educational interpreters will have responsibilities aside from just interpreting, such as bus duty or lunch duty. Full-time educational interpreters are expected to attend staff meetings, adhere to school codes of conduct, prioritize student safety, and function as a member of an educational team. They will likely also have to have background checks, as well as participate in bloodborne pathogen training, suicide awareness and prevention training, active shooter training, fire drills, and other required school trainings.

History of Deaf Education

The history of Deaf education is vast, long, and exceedingly complex (Baynton, 1996; Branson & Miller, 2002; Lane, 1984). Suffice to say, we believe it is important for educational interpreters to have a general understanding of the history of Deaf education and offer a few milestones here to help inventory evolving attitudes.

In medieval times (keep in mind there was no public education system then), Deaf people were thought of as unable to learn as speech was considered essential for thought and learning. As such, Deaf individuals were marginalized. It was in the 16th century that Pedro Ponce de León, a Spanish Benedictine monk, developed a fingerspelling technique to teach Deaf students to read, write, and speak (Abernathy, 1959; Moser et al., 1960). In the early 17th century, Juan Pablo Bonet published Ponce de León's methods (Bonet, 1620).

Fast forward to 1760 in Paris, France, where Abbé de l'Épée (in English this means Father as he was a Catholic priest) opened the first public educational institution for the Deaf, the *Institut National des jeunes sourds* de Paris. This school's approach to Deaf education was teaching academic content using *langue des signes française* (French Sign Language or LSF) and it is still open to this day.

Also in 1760, the first Deaf School in the United Kingdom opened in Scotland as the Braidwood Academy for the Deaf and Dumb. This terminology was appropriate for the time in that dumb meant a person could not speak. Now this terminology is considered a pejorative. Thomas Braidwood used a combined system of signed language, speech, and lip-reading. Braidwood moved the school to England in 1783, and after several name changes it became the Royal School for Deaf Children, which closed in 2015 after 220 years. The sign language Braidwood used in his combined system has been credited as being the precursor of modern British Sign Language (BSL) (Sutton-Spence & Woll, 1999).

In contrast, Samuel Heinicke opposed dependence on signed language and advocated teaching Deaf individuals to speak and lip-read. Heinicke opened the first oral public school for the Deaf in the world in Leipzig, Germany. In 1780, Heinicke published a book *Ueber di Denkart der Taubstummen* attacking Abbé de l'Épée. Heinicke strongly believed that sign language hindered the development of abstract thought, and that oral communication was essential for Deaf individuals to fully participate in society. He died only 12 years later, but his wife and children kept the school open, which was eventually moved to Berlin. Today, the *Sächsische Landesschule mit dem Förderschwerpunkt Hören* school uses a blended approach to teaching Deaf students but heavily emphasizes audio-verbal therapies and oral techniques.

As you can see, in this era schools for the Deaf were opening across Europe. Some used signed language, and some used oral-only education approaches, but many situated themselves in the middle by using a blended approach. However, the intense debate of oralism versus manualism was underway. (For an interesting guide through Deaf history in Europe, check out Administrator, 2014.)

Jumping ahead to 1815, Dr. Mason Cogswell, a prominent American physician with a Deaf daughter, helped set up a Deaf school in the United States. Dr. Cogswell sent Thomas Hopkins Gallaudet, a minister, to Europe to study the Braidwood methodology. The Braidwoods were unwilling to share their expertise, and Gallaudet was unconvinced the oral method was effective (Gannon, 2012; Lane, 1984; Van Cleve & Crouch, 1989).

Before leaving England, Gallaudet happened to attend a lecture by Abbé Sicard, Abbé de l'Épée's successor (l'Épée died in 1789). Two of Sicard's faculty, Laurent Clerc and Jean Massieu (both Deaf), were also in attendance. At the end of the lecture, both Clerc and Massieu invited Gallaudet to Paris to see their signed language methodology for teaching Deaf students. While in France, Gallaudet studied LSF with Clerc and convinced him to come to America for a year to establish a Deaf residential school. In 1816, Gallaudet and Clerc set sail for America, and Clerc continued to teach Gallaudet LSF and Gallaudet taught Clerc English. After 52 days, both arrived in New York and headed to Hartford, Connecticut. (You can read Clerc's journal from his journey at Disability History Museum, n.d.—*Diary of Laurent Clerc's Voyage from France to America in 1816*.)

The Connecticut Asylum for the Education and Instruction of Deaf and Dumb Persons (renamed the American School for the Deaf) opened in 1817, giving rise to the methodology of Deaf education through signed language in America. After this time, many states opened residential schools for the Deaf (Gannon, 2012).

While the debate between manualism versus oralism was intensely argued abroad, the United States was firmly rooted in signed language education for Deaf students. However, this changed in 1880 as a result of decisions made at the Second International Congress on the Education of the Deaf, hosted in Milan, Italy. Alexander Graham Bell, inventor of the telephone, argued for a complete ban on signed language at this conference (Lane, 1984). In attendance were 163 hearing delegates and one Deaf delegate (one of the five from the United States). Eight resolutions were passed which essentially declared signed language was to be banned as a method of instruction for Deaf students, and all schools in Europe switched to oral approaches to Deaf education. (You can download a copy of all those Milan speeches at IDA@Gallaudet, 2024.) The ripple effects from such a small group of people making decisions about the education of Deaf students have had far-reaching consequences. Deaf education in America was forever affected as oral-only education took hold in the late 19th and early 20th centuries. As a result, many schools for the Deaf across the United States began phasing out sign language, leading to the suppression of Deaf culture and linguistic identity. The move toward oralism marginalized Deaf educators and students, limiting their ability to communicate and learn effectively in their natural visual language (Baynton, 1996).

Leap forward to the 1960s and William Stokoe, Dorothy Casterline, and Carl Croneberg proved that ASL is a legitimate language just as any other language is. As a result of significant language planning in the 1970s, Manually Coded English (MCE) was established with several variations. These included Seeing Essential English (SEE I), Signing Exact English (SEE II), Linguistics of Visual English (LOVE), and Signed English (SE). Originally created as a tool to improve English literacy among Deaf students, MCE is not a natural language, but rather an artificially constructed system that attempts to represent spoken and written English visually.

MCE strictly follows English word order—which differs from ASL's grammar and syntax—and includes elements such as English affixes (e.g., -ing, -ed), verb tenses, articles, and prepositions that are not naturally used in ASL. To represent English vocabulary that has no direct equivalent in ASL, MCE introduces invented signs, and it often modifies existing ASL signs by adding initialization—the incorporation of the first letter of the English word into the handshape (e.g., using a V handshape for van, B for bus, T for truck). These modifications result in a system that visually mimics English rather than preserving the grammatical and cultural integrity of ASL.

By the 1980s, MCE was the dominant instructional delivery method in the United States. MCE is not a full-fledged language; although some research supports MCE use for teaching English, MCE is fundamentally poor for communicative purposes as it is inefficient and a confusing system for everyday interaction (Paul & Lee, 2010).

To date, the *Contact* between MCE and ASL forms *Contact Sign*—often incorrectly called Pidgin Signed English (PSE) (Lucas, Bayley, & Valli, 2001; Valli, Lucas, Mulrooney, & Villanueva, 2011). The underlying theme in all of these coded approaches is an artifact from the Congress of Milan and the perception of the superiority of speech over signs and, in America, of English over any other language.

As we write, we acknowledge that ASL has gained significant popularity across the United States. In fact, the Modern Languages Association (MLA) notes enrollment in ASL courses has skyrocketed, making ASL the third most studied language at colleges across the United States (Lusin, Peterson, Sulewski, & Zafer, 2023). In addition, ASL is often taught in high schools for World Language credit in many states. This shift in interest and its increasing presence in schools indicate in some ways that we are recognizing ASL as a language; however, we have not always seen this in terms of language access for Deaf students (Reagan, 2011).

Another indication of this shift toward manualism is the increasing popularity of the LEAD-K movement, which stands for Language Equality and Acquisition for Deaf Kids (LEAD-K, n.d.). In the wake of oralism, Deaf children, who are primarily born to hearing parents, are often language deprived (Arpino, 2022; Caselli, Wyatte, & Henner, 2020; Cheng, Roth, Halgren, & Mayberry, 2019; Hall, 2017; Hall, Hall, & Caselli, 2019; Hall, Levin, & Anderson, 2017). The resulting language delays have caused generations of Deaf children to start school without the language they need to participate in their education. As a result, states have begun to pass laws, known as LEAD-K legislation, to require language assessments for Deaf children from birth until at least age five (higher in some states) to ensure Deaf children are making progress in their language acquisition.

Despite the popularity of ASL and visual languages, there is still an obsession with viewing Deaf children through the medical model, which views deafness primarily as a deficit or disability. Under this model, being deaf is considered a medical condition that needs to be treated, fixed, or cured, typically through interventions like hearing aids, cochlear implants, and speech therapy so that deaf children will be "normalized."

In fact, parents are often convinced by medical professionals to embrace medical interventions and technologies (cochlear implants) and the modality of speech at the expense of language. In many cases, parents are indoctrinated to believe that hearing and speaking is better for their Deaf children rather than signing. Again, this distinction focuses on modality rather than language. Thus, the controversy between oralism and manualism still lingers in Deaf education. Regardless of what Deaf educators may believe is best for a Deaf student, many parents choose to rely solely on audio-verbal therapy to communicate with their cochlear-implanted children. We fully acknowledge our bias, as we both too often see cochlear implant and AV therapy fail, which leads to language deprivation and significant delays in all other areas (B. Cerney, 2007; Friedmann & Rusou, 2015; Geers, 2002; Geers, Mitchell, Warner-Czyz, Wang, & Eisenberg, 2017; Marschark & Hauser, 2008; Marschark, Rhoten, & Fabich, 2007; Marschark & Spencer, 2009; Reagan, 2011).

Mainstreaming of Deaf Students

Circling back to history, America saw Deaf children being moved from residential schools to local public schools in the wake of Public Law 94–142 (PL 94–142), the Education for All Handicapped Children Act. Local school districts had no idea what to do with the influx of Deaf students that were flooding their schools and no longer attending the state residential Schools for the Deaf. Educational interpreters were seen as the solution to this problem, and the need for them rose dramatically even as school districts did not know what to do with them (the educational interpreters or the students).

In the United States and Canada, staff in local school systems were (and pretty much continue to be) separated as: certified teachers, administrators (also certified teachers), and support staff (secretarial support and janitors). Federal, state, and local Offices of Special Education Services (OSES) did not exist, because all disabled students were taught in residential schools. Because of this three-category structure, most special education personnel were included within the support staff category. For example, teacher's aides (education assistants or paraprofessionals) and educational interpreters, as not-certified-teachers, were considered support staff.

Over time, as PL 94–142 morphed into the Individuals with Disabilities Education Act (IDEA), more service providers were added to the mix. It was not until 2004 that educational interpreters were officially added as Related Service Providers (McCroskey, Brafford, Reardon, Meline, & Harn, 2022). This shifted educational interpreters from the support staff category to professional related service personnel, the same category as psychologists, occupational therapists, audiologists, and speech language pathologists. Twenty years later, despite the specialized skills required to be an educational interpreter, a lack of systemic understanding of the work of educational interpreters (Fitzmaurice, 2021a) prevails and many school systems still have not moved educational interpreters out of the paraprofessional category. Despite this, we are not going to spend too much time detailing what the current system looks like; rather, we will focus on what it is supposed to be.

Direct Instruction versus Interpreted Education

There is a difference between direct instruction and an interpreted education. Direct instruction is when you and your teacher share a language and use that language as the medium of instruction. An interpreted education is when your teacher uses a different language than you, and you get your instruction through an interpreter. Several research studies show us that, no matter how skilled an interpreter is, the quality of learning that a Deaf person can achieve through an interpreter is never as great as what they can achieve through direct instruction (Cates & Delkamiller, 2021; De Meulder & Haualand, 2019; Kurz, Schick, & Hauser, 2015).

Hearing students receive direct instruction all day long. In contrast, Deaf students in mainstream classrooms, who are being taught in a language that they do not know, are not receiving direct instruction. If they need an educational interpreter, they are no longer learning through direct instruction, but through an interpreted education.

There are several factors that make an interpreted education less effective than direct instruction (Caselli, Wyatte, & Henner, 2020; Cates, 2021; Cates & Delkamiller, 2021; J. Cerney, 2007; Johnson, Taylor, Schick, Brown, & Bolster, 2018; Marschark, Sapere, Convertino, & Pelz, 2008; Marschark, Sapere, Convertino, & Seewagen, 2005; Marschark & Spencer, 2009; Schick, Williams, & Kupermintz, 2006). The first is that teachers providing direct instruction have years of education and training in their content area. Educational interpreters rarely have the same level of content knowledge as the teachers who are teaching the course. The second factor is that interpretations are just that—interpretations. The process of interpreting involves making choices about meaning, intent, and importance that influence how the recipient of the interpretation perceives the message (Roy, 2000; Russell, 2002; Wadensjö, 1998). Time plays a significant factor in the quality of interpreter processing because simultaneous interpreting does not allow time for detailed analysis of the source message. Another factor is the difference between Deaf and hearing student instructional needs. A lesson that is designed for hearing students and interpreted to Deaf students does not take into account the ways that Deaf students learn best (Hall et al., 2019; Humphries et al., 2016; Mayberry, 2002). It also does not take into account language, or language features, that the Deaf student may not be familiar with. It does not take into account the effects of language deprivation, information deprivation, and the different lived experiences of Deaf and hearing students. Therefore, the lesson is less likely to be accessible in its entirety to a Deaf student than to a hearing student, even when interpreted into ASL by a qualified professional (Kurz, 2012; Kurz, Schick, & Hauser, 2015).

Ideally, when a qualified teacher of the Deaf is teaching Deaf students in ASL, they are able to take these myriad factors into account in their instruction. This approach is much more effective at meeting the needs of Deaf students than a lesson that is designed for hearing students (Cates & Delkamiller, 2021; Kurz, Schick, & Hauser, 2015). This is true whether students are on grade level or receiving special education support services due to academic delays in specific content areas.

In educational settings, you may hear teachers refer to instruction as "direct instruction" when it is one-on-one. However, even if a special education teacher is providing one-on-one instruction to a Deaf child, if they are using an interpreter, it is not direct instruction. If an educational interpreter is providing an interpretation of the material, that is considered interpreted instruction (Kurz, 2012; Kurz, Schick, & Hauser, 2015).

Truly, mainstreaming remains a 50-year social experiment with dismal outcomes for Deaf students. All the research indicates that direct instruction in self-contained programs or residential schools leads to better outcomes for Deaf students (Anglin-Jaffe, 2020; Cates & Delkamiller, 2021; De Meulder & Haualand, 2019; Levesque & Duncan, 2024). An interpreted education is not the best bet, but certainly is common practice, so let's dive in!

Job Titles and Status of Educational Interpreters

We recognize job titles of educational interpreters vary greatly around the United States. Here, we use the job title "educational interpreter" to refer to anyone providing access (i.e., interpreting) in a school system (National Association of Interpreters in Education, 2019). While some school systems use different job titles, we consider the term "educational interpreter" to be the best choice. In some cases, educational interpreters are incorrectly categorized as paraprofessionals and systemically subordinate to teachers. Positioning educational interpreters in this way is detrimental to the profession and to the students who rely on these services, particularly since it may confuse the roles occupied by these professionals.

The role of an educational interpreter should not be confused with that of a paraprofessional or educational assistant. While educational assistants often perform supportive tasks and have a subordinate role in the educational setting, educational interpreters have distinct responsibilities and ascribe to professional standards. Unlike paraprofessionals, educational interpreters are specialized professionals with specific training and credentials in interpreting, focusing on providing language and content access for Deaf students in their educational environment. In this volume, we recognize the current status of educational interpreters, but we also highlight best practices of how these professionals can and should be integrated into the educational system to optimally provide language access.

Summary

The chapter explores the differences between interpreting for adults and interpreting for Deaf children with emerging language skills. It also reviews the historical and legislative background that has shaped educational interpreting. This chapter also defines educational interpreters as professionals and explores the history of Deaf education as it has evolved over centuries, beginning with early methods of teaching Deaf individuals through signed language and oral techniques. Key historical milestones include the development of signed language methods to the opening of the American School for the Deaf. The chapter notes that a significant shift in Deaf education occurred at the Milan Conference (1880) when the conference endorsed oralism and ultimately pushed signed language aside in many schools. Despite this, ASL gained recognition as a legitimate language in the 1960s.

From there, we discussed the Education for All Handicapped Children Act of 1975, which led to mainstreaming Deaf students into regular schools, increasing the need for educational interpreters. Initially viewed as support staff, educational interpreters were later recognized as related service providers alongside professionals like psychologists and speech language pathologists. However, many schools still incorrectly categorize them as paraprofessionals.

This chapter also discussed interpreted versus direct instruction. Deaf students experiencing an interpreted education receive lessons designed for hearing students that are interpreted into ASL. Research indicates that this is less effective than direct instruction by a teacher fluent in ASL. Interpreted education may fail to fully meet Deaf students' needs, especially when educational interpreters lack the content knowledge of the teachers they are interpreting for.

Finally, this chapter discussed position titles and the overall status of educational interpreters as professionals with specialized training, distinct from paraprofessionals or educational assistants, and we argue they should be recognized as such in school systems.

Thought Questions

1 How has the historical marginalization of signed languages continued to influence the way educational interpreters are viewed and used in today's school systems?
2 How did the debate between oralism and manualism impact Deaf education in Europe and the United States?
3 What role did the Second International Congress on the Education of the Deaf play in shaping Deaf education, and how did it influence educational practices?
4 Why was the validation of ASL as a true human language in the 1960s such a big deal?
5 How did the introduction of Manually Coded English (MCE) in the 1970s affect Deaf education, and what are its strengths and limitations?
6 What changes occurred in the role and recognition of educational interpreters following the passage of the Education for All Handicapped Children Act (PL 94–142) and the Individuals with Disabilities Education Act (IDEA)?
7 If you could go back in time to the Second International Congress on the Education of the Deaf with all of the research we have to date, what argument would you present at the Congress in support of manualism?

References

Abernathy, E. R. (1959). An historical sketch of the manual alphabets. *American Annals of the Deaf*, 104(2), 232–240.

Administrator. (2014). Deaf history - Europe. Deafhistory.eu. https://www.deafhistory.eu.

Anglin-Jaffe, H. (2020). Isolation and aspiration: Deaf adults reflect on the educational legacy of special schooling. *British Educational Research Journal*, 46(6), 1468–1486.

Arpino, K. (2022). *Starved for knowledge: The effect of language deprivation and "mainstream" education on deaf accessibility to the United States education system.* Honors Scholar Theses. 861. https://opencommons.uconn.edu/srhonors_theses/861.

Baynton, D. C. (1996). *Forbidden signs: American culture and the campaign against sign language*. Chicago, IL: University of Chicago Press.

Bonet, J. P. (1620). *Reduction de las letras y arte para enseñar a ablar los mudos*. Madrid: Francisco Abarca de Angulo.

Branson, J., & Miller, D. (2002). *Damned for their difference: The cultural construction of deaf people as "disabled"*. Washington, DC: Gallaudet University Press.

Caselli, N., Wyatte, H., & Henner, J. (2020). American Sign Language interpreters in public schools: An illusion of inclusion that perpetuates language deprivation. *Maternal and Child Health Journal*, 24(11), 1323–1329.

Cates, D. (2021). Patterns in EIPA test scores and implications for interpreter education. *Journal of Interpretation*, 29(1), 6.

Cates, D., & Delkamiller, J. (2021). The impact of sign language interpreter skill on education outcomes in K–12 settings. In E. Winston & S. B. Fitzmaurice (Eds.), *Advances in Educational Interpreting* (pp. 19–30). Washington, DC: Gallaudet University Press.

Cerney, B. (2007). Language acquisition, language teaching, and the interpreter as a model for language input. http://www.handandmind.org/LgAcquisition.pdf.

Cerney, J. (2007). *Deaf education in America: Voices of children from inclusion settings*. Washington, DC: Gallaudet University Press.

Cheng, Q., Roth, A., Halgren, E., & Mayberry, R. I. (2019). Effects of early language deprivation on brain connectivity: Language pathways in deaf native and late first-language learners of American Sign Language. *Frontiers in Human Neuroscience*, 13, 1–12.

Child Welfare Information Gateway. (2023). Mandatory reporting of child abuse and neglect. Washington, DC: U.S. Department of Health and Human Services, Administration for Children and Families, Children's Bureau. https://www.childwelfare.gov/resources/mandatory-reporting-child-abuse-and-neglect/.

De Meulder, M., & Haualand, H. (2019). Sign language interpreting services: A quick fix for inclusion? *Translation and Interpreting Studies*, 16(1), 19–40.

Department of Education. (2001). Education white paper 6: special needs education – Building an inclusive education and training system. Pretoria: Department of Education. https://www.gov.za/sites/default/files/gcis_document/201409/educ61.pdf.

Department for Education & Department of Health. (2015). *Special educational needs and disability code of practice: 0 to 25 years (Statutory guidance for organisations which work with and support children and young people who have special educational needs or disabilities)*. https://www.gov.uk/government/publications/send-code-of-practice-0-to-25.

Disability History Museum. (n.d.). *Diary of Laurent Clerc's voyage from France to America in 1816*. https://www.disabilitymuseum.org/dhm/lib/detail.html?id=687&page=all.

Fitzmaurice, S. (2017). Unregulated autonomy: Uncredentialed educational interpreters in rural schools. *American Annals of the Deaf*, 162(3), 253–264.

Fitzmaurice, S. B. (2021a). *The role of the educational interpreter: Perceptions of administrators and teachers*. Washington, DC: Gallaudet University Press.

Fitzmaurice, S. B. (2021b). There is no I(nterpreter) in your team. In E. Winston & S. B. Fitzmaurice (Eds.), *Advances in educational interpreting* (pp. 336–351). Washington, DC: Gallaudet University Press.

Fitzmaurice, S. B. (2021c). The realistic role metaphor for educational interpreters. In E. Winston & S. B. Fitzmaurice (Eds.), *Advances in educational interpreting* (pp. 285–307). Washington, DC: Gallaudet University Press.

Friedmann, N., & Rusou, D. (2015). Critical period for first language: The crucial role of language input during the first year of life. *Current Opinion in Neurobiology*, 35, 27–34.

Gannon, J. R. (2012). *Deaf heritage: A narrative history of deaf America* (7th ed.). National Association of the Deaf.

Geers, A. (2002). Factors affecting the development of speech, language, and literacy in children with early cochlear implantation. *Language, Speech, and Hearing Services in the School*, 33(3), 172–183.

Geers, A. E., Mitchell, C. M., Warner-Czyz, A., Wang, N.-Y., & Eisenberg, L. S. (2017). Early sign language exposure and cochlear implantation benefits. *Pediatrics*, 140(1), e20163489.

Government of British Columbia. (1996). School Act [RSBC 1996] Chapter 412. https://www.bclaws.gov.bc.ca/civix/document/id/complete/statreg/96412_00.

Government of Canada. (1982). *Canadian Charter of Rights and Freedoms*. https://laws-lois.justice.gc.ca/eng/const/page-15.html.

Government of Ontario. (1990). *Education Act, R.S.O.* 1990, c. E.2. https://www.ontario.ca/laws/statute/90e02.

Hall, M. L., Hall, W. C., & Caselli, N. K. (2019). Deaf children need language, not (just) speech. *First Language*, 39(4), 367–395.

Hall, W. C. (2017). What you don't know can hurt you: The risk of language deprivation by impairing sign language development in deaf children. *Maternal and Child Health Journal*, 21(5), 961–965.

Hall, W. C., Levin, L. L., & Anderson, M. L. (2017). Language deprivation syndrome: A possible neurodevelopmental disorder with sociocultural origins. *Social Psychiatry and Psychiatric Epidemiology*, 52(6), 761–776.

Humphries, T., Kushalnagar, P., Mathur, G., Napoli, D. J., Padden, C., Rathmann, C., & Smith, S. R. (2016). Language acquisition for deaf children: Reducing the harms of zero tolerance to the use of alternative approaches. *Harm Reduction Journal*, 13(1): 16.

IDA@Gallaudet. (2024). *Report of the Proceedings of the International Congress on the Education of the Deaf, held at Milan, September 6th-11th, 1880*. London: W.H. Allen & Co. https://ida.gallaudet.edu/deaf_rare_books/107/.

Johnson, L., Taylor, M., Schick, B., Brown, S., & Bolster, L. (2018). *Complexities in educational interpreting: An investigation into patterns of practice*. Edmonton: Interpreting Consolidated.

Kurz, C. A. (2012). Using direct instruction to teach mathematics to students with moderate to severe disabilities. *Journal of Deaf Studies and Deaf Education*, 17(4), 476–488.

Kurz, K. B., Schick, B., & Hauser, P. C. (2015). Deaf children's science content learning in direct instruction versus interpreted instruction. *Journal of Science Education for Students with Disabilities*, 18(1), 23–37.

Lane, H. (1984). *When the mind hears: A history of the deaf*. New York: Random House.

Lawson, H. R. (2021). Educational interpreters: Facilitating communication or facilitating education? In E. A. Winston & S. B. Fitzmaurice (Eds.), *Advances in educational interpreting* (pp. 245–265). Washington, DC: Gallaudet University Press.

LEAD-K. (n.d.). Language Equality and Acquisition for Deaf Kids. Retrieved April 28, 2025, from https://www.lead-k.org.

Levesque, E., & Duncan, J. (2024). Inclusive education for deaf students: Pass or fail. *Deafness & Education International*, 26(2), 125–126.

Lucas, C., Bayley, R., & Valli, C. (2001). *Sociolinguistic variation in American Sign Language*. Washington, DC: Gallaudet University Press.

Lusin, N., Peterson, T., Sulewski, C., & Zafer, R. (2023). *Enrollments in languages other than English in US institutions of higher education*. New York: Modern Languages Association.

Marschark, M., & Hauser, P. (2008). Cognitive underpinnings of learning by deaf and hard of hearing students: Differences, diversity, and directions. In M. Marschark & P. Hauser (Eds), *Deaf cognition: Foundations and outcomes* (pp. 3–23). New York: Oxford University Press.

Marschark, M., Rhoten, C., & Fabich, M. (2007). Effects of cochlear implants on children's reading and academic achievement. *Journal of Deaf Studies and Deaf Education*, 12(3), 269–282.

Marschark, M., Sapere, P., Convertino, C. M., & Pelz, J. (2008). Learning via direct and mediated instruction by deaf students. *The Journal of Deaf Studies and Deaf Education*, 13(4), 546–561.

Marschark, M., Sapere, P., Convertino, C., & Seewagen, R. (2005). Access to post-secondary education through sign language interpreting. *The Journal of Deaf Studies and Deaf Education*, 10(1), 38–50.

Marschark, M., & Spencer, P. E. (2009). *Evidence of best practice models and outcomes in the education of deaf and hard-of-hearing children: An international review*. Trim: National Council for Special Education.

Mayberry, R. I. (2002). Cognitive development in deaf children: The interface of language and perception in neuropsychology. *Handbook of Neuropsychology*, 8, 71–107.

McCroskey, C., Brafford, T., Reardon, K., Meline, M., & Harn, B. (2022). IDEA: History and legal issues. Routledge Resources Online – Education. Abingdon: Routledge. doi:10.4324/9781138609877-REE155-1.

Moser, H. M., O'Neill, J. J., Oyer, H. J., Wolfe, S. M., Abernathy, E. A., & Schowe Jr, B. M. (1960). Historical aspects of manual communication. *Journal of Speech and Hearing Disorders*, 25(2), 145–151.

National Association of Interpreters in Education. (2019). Professional guidelines for interpreting in educational settings (1st ed.). Retrieved from www.naiedu.org/guidelines.

Paul, P. V., & Lee, C. (2010). *Deaf and hard of hearing students' language, literacy, and academic development*. London: Pearson.

Reagan, T. (2011). Ideological barriers to American Sign Language: Unpacking linguistic resistance. *Sign Language Studies*, 11(4), 606–636.

Republic of South Africa. (1996). *South African Schools Act 84 of 1996*. https://www.gov.za/documents/south-african-schools-act.

Roy, C. B. (2000). *Interpreting as a discourse process*. New York: Oxford University Press.

Russell, D. (2002). Interpreter interaction in educational settings: A look at deaf students and interpreters. *Sign Language Studies*, 3(2), 183–216.

Schick, B., Williams, K., & Kupermintz, H. (2006). Look who's being left behind: Educational interpreters and access to education for deaf and hard-of-hearing students. *The Journal of Deaf Studies and Deaf Education*, 11(1), 3–20.

Sutton-Spence, R., & Woll, B. (1999). *The linguistics of British Sign Language: An introduction*. Cambridge: Cambridge University Press.

United Kingdom Government. (2014). *Children and Families Act 2014*. https://www.legislation.gov.uk/ukpga/2014/6/contents/enacted.

Valli, C., Lucas, C., Mulrooney, K. J., & Villanueva, M. (2011). *Linguistics of American Sign Language: An introduction* (5th ed.). Washington, DC: Gallaudet University Press.

Van Cleve, J. V., & Crouch, B. A. (1989). *A place of their own: Creating the Deaf community in America*. Washington, DC: Gallaudet University Press.

Wadensjö, C. (1998). *Interpreting as interaction*. London: Longman.

3 The System, Constituents, and Stakeholders

The education of Deaf students in the United States is shaped by a complex interplay of legal mandates, pedagogical philosophies, and systemic structures that often fail to fully account for the linguistic and cultural experiences of Deaf individuals. Since the passage of the Individuals with Disabilities Education Act (IDEA), the majority of Deaf students have been placed in mainstream public schools, where they typically rely on sign language interpreters for access to instruction and peer interaction. However, access is not synonymous with equity. Educational interpreters must navigate far more than just language—they operate within systems that frequently misunderstand or undervalue their roles, while simultaneously supporting students whose communication needs are often marginalized or misunderstood. This chapter examines the critical position of the educational interpreter, the structural realities of Deaf Education (Deaf Ed), and the importance of centering Deaf perspectives in efforts to create truly inclusive, language-rich learning environments.

The Education System

Since the implementation of IDEA as Public Law 94–142 (Individuals with Disabilities Education Act, 20 U.S.C. § 1400 et seq., 2004) children with disabilities have been regularly educated alongside their non-disabled peers. For Deaf students, this means they are predominantly no longer educated in state residential schools for the Deaf, but rather mainstreamed into their neighborhood public schools. This practice resulted in the birth of educational interpreting and the rapid decline in attendance at residential Schools for the Deaf, many of which have since closed. To date, several sources report that over 85%–90% of Deaf students attend regular public schools—many navigating their education by way of an educational interpreter (Knoors & Marschark, 2014; National Association of the Deaf, n.d.; National Deaf Center on Postsecondary Outcomes, 2018; LaPlante, 2023).

The education system itself has many different levels. In the United States, the largest is the United States Department of Education, which oversees general federal-level education policies and programs (such as IDEA), regulation, civil rights enforcement in education, data collection, and funding/grants.

DOI: 10.4324/9781003423058-3

Different states call them by different names; however, the next major level is the State Department of Education (SDE). SDEs are generally responsible for the public education in their respective states. They do this by setting standards for curriculum, assessments, resource allocation, educator certification, school safety, and Special Education (SPED) services. Some SDEs oversee regional SPED programs that serve multiple local education agencies. These regional programs have different names in different states, but they are generally responsible for supporting school districts in the education of students with disabilities. Educational interpreter services sometimes fall under the purview of these regional programs.

Local Education Agencies (LEA), or school districts (also called by different names in different states), are the next layer in this complex system. LEAs are groups of several different schools—for example elementary, middle, high school—and can be very large with multiple schools for each level, or so small that they have one single school building for all students PK-12. LEAs are charged with implementing the curriculum determined by the state, managing personnel and facilities, etc.

From there, we have public schools themselves which consist of administrators (principals, vice principals), teachers (both general education teachers and SPED teachers), Related Service Providers (such as speech language pathologists, psychologists, occupational therapists, physical therapists, and educational interpreters), and support staff (such as nurses, counselors, media specialists, paraprofessionals, administrative staff, custodial staff, food service workers, etc.). Naturally, the smallest unit is the individual classroom, of which there are many! Figure 3.1 showcases these levels.

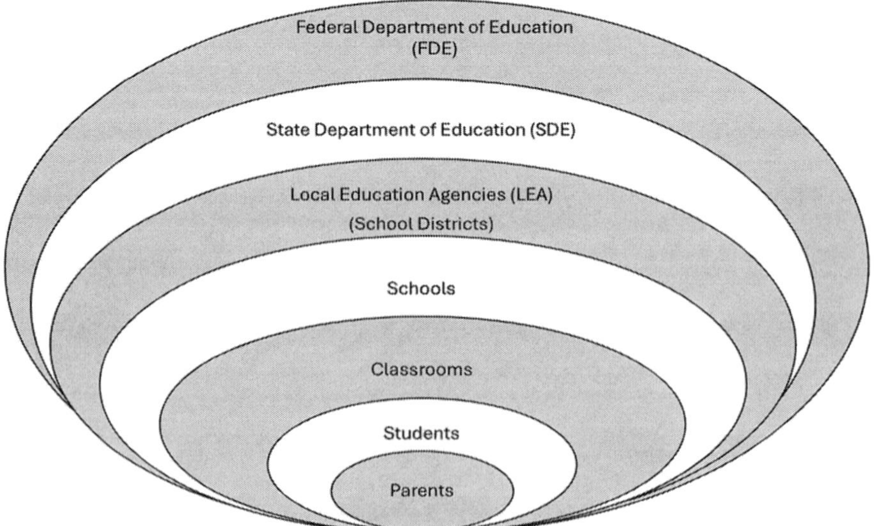

Figure 3.1 Levels of the Education System

What is absent in the education system are Deaf communities themselves. Despite being the primary stakeholders in Deaf Ed (many of whom have the lived experience of mainstreamed Deaf Ed), Deaf individuals continue to be excluded from major decisions regarding Deaf Ed. Members of the Deaf community are often not invited to IEP meetings for Deaf students as individuals with special knowledge regarding the Deaf child. This is because of a combination of systemic bias, misunderstanding of Deaf expertise, and structural barriers within the education system. Despite advocacy efforts by organizations such as the National Association of the Deaf emphasizing the principle of "Nothing About Us Without Us," Deaf professionals remain underrepresented in school leadership and educational policymaking, and Deaf community members are absent from the education system (Individuals with Disabilities Education Act, 2004; Lane, 1992; National Association of the Deaf, n.d.).

Now that we have an idea of what the multifaceted education system comprises, it is important to understand how that system uses language.

Deaf Ed vs SPED

The education system in the United States primarily uses a deficit view of deafness. Thus, the approach of the majority of educators is going to be auditory habilitation of Deaf children, rather than focusing on the holistic language needs, including visual language needs, of Deaf children. Under this view, a child may experience difficulties in their education at the fault of their deafness as opposed to the fault of a system that is inaccessible to them. We explore each of these concepts in greater depth in later chapters, but it is important when framing a conversation of the education system to recognize that it is not built for Deaf children.

The education system as a whole is not designed to teach a child their first language. An unspoken assumption in education is that a child comes to school with a language. In SPED, this assumption holds true. Most children who come into SPED already have some functional first language, though there are certain disabilities that cause underdeveloped language, leading to a focus on the use of functional communication devices with children who have such disabilities. However, most Deaf students come into the education system with an incomplete grasp of their first language, not because of an inherent language disorder, but because of language deprivation. Therefore, Deaf Ed is more focused on supporting a child's access to language than SPED is.

However, the philosophical differences between oralist approaches and manualist approaches to education result in the focus being placed on auditory habilitation for most Deaf children. Some state legislation, such as LEAD-K, as well as the drafted Alice Cogswell Macy Act, aims to combat the effects of a medical or auditory-focused, deficit approach to deafness. This legislation aims to center language access as the critical issue in early childhood development for Deaf children.

It is possible for a Deaf student to receive services from a teacher of the Deaf but no services from a SPED teacher, or a student may receive services from both. In most systems, Deaf Ed is housed under SPED. Next, we discuss the similarities and differences between SPED and Deaf Ed philosophies and practices.

Similarities

SPED and Deaf Ed both serve students who have disabilities. Therefore, it is not unusual for Deaf students to have an IEP (Individuals with Disabilities Education Act, 2004), a 504 plan (Rehabilitation Act of 1973), interpreter services, or other accessibility services provided as a result of their rights under the Americans with Disabilities Act (ADA) (1990). In the *Perez v. Sturgis* (2023) case, the Supreme Court found that school systems can be held accountable for the provision of *qualified* interpreters under the ADA, and that due process under IDEA does not exempt a school from their obligations under the ADA. Students served by both SPED and Deaf Ed programs undeniably have ADA rights that schools are responsible for meeting in addition to their educational needs.

Deaf students who are also receiving SPED services may be served by both a teacher of the Deaf and a SPED teacher, or a teacher who has endorsements to teach both SPED and Deaf Ed. As an educational interpreter, you will work with both SPED and Deaf Ed teachers over the course of your career. Most of the time when you are interpreting for a Deaf Ed teacher, it will be because they have not learned ASL even though they teach Deaf children (Guardino, 2015; Supporting Success for Children with Hearing Loss, 2024; Swanepoel & Störbeck, 2022). Regardless of your personal philosophy, it is important to maintain a respectful, collegial relationship with the teachers with whom you work in order to ensure effective services for Deaf students.

It is common for SPED teachers to want to learn some sign language to communicate directly with Deaf students. Many will pick up some conversational language but cannot teach academic content in ASL. It is a tricky situation to navigate as an interpreter when working with a teacher who wants to use ASL with the student directly but does not have the language to produce a coherent, grammatically accurate message. Therefore, you may find yourself in an awkward situation where the SPED teacher is attempting to sign for themselves during instruction but is signing inaccurately. It is important to learn how to navigate those conversations to support the SPED teacher's desire to learn to communicate directly with their students while ensuring that the Deaf student can access their education. It may help to suggest that they sign directly with the student about conversational topics, but allow you to interpret during instruction time.

Differences

SPED and Deaf Ed have different foundational assumptions. In SPED, the foundational assumption is that a student has some type of disability that has resulted in a gap between their performance in an educational setting and that of their same-aged peers. The disability may be physical, mental, social, emotional, or behavioral.

In SPED, there is also an assumption that students have some kind of language foundation. There may be an expectation of specific language disabilities, such as for a child with a language processing disorder, but it is unlikely for teachers going into SPED to assume that most of their student population will lack a native, or first, language.

Another foundational assumption of SPED is that students will need *specially designed instruction* (SDI) to be able to close achievement gaps between their performance level and their expected grade level. The goal of SPED is to provide this instruction at their home school district with as little time removed from the general education setting as possible. Removal from the general education setting is considered *restrictive* (where the concept of *Least Restrictive Environment* comes from). The idea of sending all students with a particular disability to one place to be educated together is an anathema to SPED. In fact, from a SPED lens, a Deaf school would be seen as one of the most restrictive environments for a Deaf student, second only to a locked facility.

In Deaf Ed, the foundational assumption is that the child is going to need access to communication or language, depending on the philosophical approach of the educator (Lane, 1999; Marschark & Hauser, 2012). The philosophical differences between educating Deaf students using oralist approaches versus bilingual approaches result in a substantial difference in focal areas for Deaf Ed programs. It is common for teachers of the Deaf to have coursework in audiology and speech language pathology, as well as instructional methods for Deaf students. However, ASL fluency is not a standard requirement in Deaf Ed programs. As an educational interpreter, you may end up interpreting for instruction time with the teacher of the Deaf (Swanepoel & Störbeck, 2022).

Since deafness is considered a low-incidence disability, many school districts have only one or two Deaf students. It is common for Deaf students in these types of mainstream settings to receive services from an *itinerant teacher*. An itinerant teacher is one who works with multiple students across multiple school buildings. It is highly unlikely a school district will hire a full-time teacher of the Deaf for just one or two students, so itinerant teachers serve multiple districts or school buildings to spread the cost of their services. This happens regardless of the number of minutes of direct instruction a Deaf child needs for a Free and Appropriate Public Education (FAPE). Furthermore, as we previously discussed, not all teachers of the Deaf are fluent enough to provide direct instruction in ASL.

Some school districts engage in the practice of *cluster sites*, which is when the district identifies one single school for all Deaf children to attend, regardless of which school is considered their home school. While this practice creates a critical mass of Deaf students for the benefits of socialization and centralizing resources, it has been challenged in courts as a violation of the child's right to be educated at their neighborhood school.

There are also differences in the curricular focus for SPED and Deaf Ed services. SPED typically focuses on core curriculum, whereas Deaf Ed often also focuses on the *Expanded Core Curriculum for the Deaf and Hard of Hearing* (Colorado Department of Education, 2014). As a result of these curricular differences, many teachers of the Deaf do not do direct instruction in core content areas, though they may provide specially designed instruction in core areas as part of IEP goals.

The Individualized Education Program (IEP)

States have different terms they use for labeling SPED qualifications including "exceptionality," "disability," "eligibility," "diagnosis," and "verification." These all refer to the reason why the child is eligible for SPED services. When a school suspects a child has a disability, the school district has 60 days to complete evaluations before holding a disability suspect meeting to determine the child's eligibility for SPED services. This initial process is known as "child find" and the disability suspect meeting is called a multidisciplinary team meeting (MDT). If the result of the MDT is that the child is eligible for SPED services, an Individualized Education Program (IEP) is established for the child. (*Note it is a program, not a plan. Many people are apt to make this error.*) If the child does not have an educational need resulting from their disability, the school may establish a 504 Plan. IEPs are governed by IDEA, whereas 504 Plans are governed by Section 504 of the Rehabilitation Act.

There are procedural, substantive, and implementation requirements in place for IEPs. To be in compliance with federal law, school districts must ensure IEPs satisfy these requirements. Procedural requirements deal with how, where, and when an IEP is developed (i.e., how children are identified and evaluated, how parents are involved in the process, how due process complaints are handled, who must be involved in developing an IEP, and what components are necessary to include in an IEP). Substantive requirements deal with the content of the IEP (i.e., a statement of the *Present Level of Academic Achievement and Functional Performance* (PLAAFP), measurable goals for all identified areas of need in the PLAAFP, and how progress monitoring will be conducted).

According to two major US Supreme Court cases, *Board of Education of the Hendrick Hudson Central School District v. Rowley* and *Endrew F. v. Douglas County School District Re-1*, the substance of the IEP must ensure a child can make appropriate educational progress given their circumstances (Board of Education of the Hendrick Hudson Central School District v. Rowley, 1982; Endrew F. v. Douglas County School District Re-1, 2017). Implementation requirements deal with how the parts of the IEP are carried out (i.e., ensuring all service minutes are met, that progress monitoring is completed).

IEPs detail a student's goals, services, activities, and accommodations. Academic goals are often in the areas of reading, writing, and/or math. Social emotional goals are often in the areas of self-advocacy and pragmatic development for Deaf students, often aligning with the *Expanded Core Curriculum for*

Students who are Deaf or Hard of Hearing (Iowa Department of Education, 2019). Each goal will state where the child is currently performing and what their target is for the academic year, as well as giving a statement of progress monitoring, or how their work toward the goal is measured during the year and who is responsible for reporting on it. These goals are important for the educational interpreter to know because the goals will help them understand the student's educational needs. In fact, students may have goals around the use of their educational interpreter as well.

Services and accommodations are what the student needs in order to meet their goals and receive a FAPE. Services in an IEP are always detailed with a number of minutes per day, week, or month that a child receives the service. If a child has an educational interpreter, this generally means that their service minutes are every school day, all day. A school is required to meet all of the service minutes as detailed in the IEP. Therefore, if the child has an educational interpreter who is absent for some reason, the school must provide a substitute sign language interpreter. Not all school districts can provide substitutes on short notice, so it is a good idea for there to be a substitute plan in the IEP for occasions when the educational interpreter is absent and a sub is unavailable.

Services are usually tied to goals. However, some services, such as educational interpreting, may not have a particular goal tied to them. For a child on an IEP, goals and services must be reviewed annually and can be amended at any time. If a child meets their goals, they may be exited from their IEP. Qualification for SPED must be verified every three years. At this time, the team does a comprehensive review, including psychological testing, to ensure that the child is receiving appropriate SPED services. Deaf children who do not qualify for SPED services or who are exited from an IEP will still qualify for a 504 Plan for accommodations.

504 Plans

A 504 Plan is for students with disabilities who require accommodations to access their education, such as closed captioning, interpreters, and note-takers (Rehabilitation Act of 1973). An IEP is specifically for students who also qualify for SPED services based on having an identified educational need resulting from a disability (Individuals with Disabilities Education Act, 2004).

It is critical that educational interpreters understand the difference between an accommodation and a modification. Accommodations change how a student accesses the curriculum, but do not change what curriculum they are learning. Modifications change what the student is learning. A 504 Plan may change how the child accesses their education, but it does not change what they learn. An IEP may change what the student learns through curriculum modifications, how the student learns through accommodations, or both. Regardless of the type of plan a Deaf child has, if they have an educational interpreter, the interpreter has valuable insight to contribute to the team. A summary of the differences between IEPs and 504 Plans is given in Table 3.1.

Table 3.1 Differences between 504 and IEP Plans

504 Plans	*IEP Plans*
Governing Law	Governing Law
• Section 504 of the Rehabilitation Act	• Individuals with Disabilities Education Act (IDEA)
Requirement to Qualify	Requirement to Qualify
• Identified disability that requires accommodations to access the general education curriculum	• Identified educational need resulting from a disability that requires specially designed instruction
Required Team Members	Required Team Members
• Parent • Child (when appropriate) • General Education Teacher • School Administrator • School 504 Plan Coordinator • Person qualified to interpret evaluation results • By invitation, others with specialized expertise or knowledge of the child	• Parent • Child (when appropriate) • General Education Teacher (if applicable) • Special Education Teacher • School Administrator • Person qualified to interpret evaluation results • By invitation, others with specialized expertise or knowledge of the child
Plan Components	Plan Components
• Accommodations and supports child needs to access the general education curriculum	• Child's present level of performance • Measurable annual goal(s) • How the child will participate in standardized assessments • Accommodations and supports child needs • How the child will participate in general education and special education • Related services • Extended School Year (ESY) • Transition plan to post-high school (for high school students or those at age 16) • Special factors
Timeline for Review	Timeline for Review
• Annual	• Annual review of goals • Triannual reevaluation to qualify

The IEP Team: Related Service Providers

Educational interpreters are Related Service Providers according to IDEA Section 300.34. Related Service Providers (Individuals with Disabilities Education Act, 2004) are personnel who provide specialized support or services to a child in SPED. They are generally invited to participate in a child's IEP because they have special expertise and knowledge of the child. Each member of the IEP Team serves a different role and function. The most common Related Service Providers working with Deaf students are Teachers of the Deaf, audiologists, speech language pathologists (SLPs), and educational interpreters. For children with additional identified disabilities, there may be other service providers on their IEP. These other service providers may include occupational therapists (OTs), physical therapists (PTs), and nurses or other medical personnel.

Teachers of the Deaf

In general, teachers of the Deaf are responsible for ensuring that Deaf students are receiving education specific to their deafness. According to the Council for Exceptional Children (n.d.), a teacher of the Deaf should have training in individual learning differences, learning environments, curriculum content, assessment, instructional strategies, ethical practices, collaboration, programs, services, and outcomes. However, not all teachers of the Deaf serve the same function, and not all teachers of the Deaf are fluent in ASL (Alawajee, 2022; Beal-Alvarez & Scheetz, 2015; Luckner & Ayantoye, 2013).

There are different types of teachers of the Deaf: early childhood education teachers, Deaf school or center-based teachers, co-teachers, itinerant teachers, and teacher consultants. Early childhood education teachers work with families and in preschool settings. Their primary focus is on social language development and pre-literacy skills. Deaf school or center-based teachers of the Deaf provide direct instruction in classrooms with all Deaf students. Center-based teachers usually have classrooms in public schools and support the needs of Deaf students in the broader general education environment. Co-teachers work side-by-side with general education or SPED teachers to provide specialist instruction for Deaf students in a larger mainstream environment. Itinerant teachers of the Deaf generally have caseloads of students across multiple schools or districts. They provide consultation to other service providers and some specialized instruction to students as designated on student IEPs.

Deaf students with itinerant teachers of the Deaf are usually mainstreamed with hearing students in SPED and/or general education classes for most of their school day. The itinerant model is quite popular in areas with smaller numbers of Deaf students insufficient to support a center-based program. However, this results in fewer hours of direct instruction opportunities for these students, especially if they are learning primarily through ASL (Luckner & Ayantoye, 2013). Educational interpreters are beneficial for providing access, but they cannot replace the benefit of direct instruction from qualified teachers of the Deaf.

Audiologists

The audiologist is responsible for identifying and explaining the child's hearing levels and what they can or cannot hear. The audiologist is also responsible for ensuring that the child has appropriate hearing assistive technology (HAT) equipment, if they use it. This includes hearing aids, cochlear implants, frequency modulation/digital modulation (FM/DM) systems, and other types of HAT that support the child's hearing. Educational audiologists are a special type of audiologist; they support students in educational settings as part of the IEP or 504 Plan team. They provide services above and beyond those of audiologists in private clinics (Educational Audiology Association, 2019).

Speech Language Pathologists

The speech language pathologist (SLP) is responsible for working on any goals related to speech, articulation, or language comprehension or production. They specialize in speech and language disorders. Most SLPs are not trained to work specifically with students who are deaf or hard of hearing. In order to support a child's ASL development, an SLP would need to be fluent in ASL themselves. As most are not, educational interpreters may support the SLP in their work with Deaf students, particularly with language-related goals. If an SLP is working with a Deaf student on Visual Phonics (a system of visual cues designed to represent speech sounds), the interpreter may need to learn this system to use it during classroom reading instruction (Waddy-Smith & Wilson, 2003). In this way, the interpreter carries the work of the SLP beyond the pull-out sessions and integrates it into the school day.

Teachers

The general education teacher is responsible for core classroom content. They are also responsible for implementing any accommodations included in the child's IEP. Common accommodations for Deaf students include "preferential seating" (usually at the front of the room which, ironically, is not what many Deaf people prefer), copies of teacher slides/notes, closed captioning, use of personal FM or DM microphones, and extended time on tests. Teachers are also responsible for classroom discipline.

The SPED teacher is responsible for providing specially designed instruction in the area of the child's IEP goals. They may do this through push-in services where they provide materials and support to the general education teacher, pull-out services where they work one-on-one or in small groups with students, or a combination of both.

Administrators

School administrators must be present at IEP meetings because they have authority to approve costs associated with the IEP. Costs generally include specialized personnel, such as interpreters, and resources such as transportation (Fitzmaurice, 2021). It is common for larger school districts to be able to hire their own teachers of the Deaf, educational interpreters, SLPs, and other Related Service Providers. Smaller school districts often receive SPED services through regional programs or services. These regional programs or services have different names in different states, so be sure to identify what they are called in your state.

IEP Team Meetings

Often, educational interpreters are asked to interpret IEP meetings for participating students, or for a child's Deaf parents. Educational interpreters need to pay careful attention to their state's licensing regulations because they may not be allowed to interpret for Deaf adults based on the type of qualifications they have to work in their state. In any case, it is always best practice to have an outside interpreter interpret IEP meetings while the child's regular educational interpreter attends the IEP meeting. Thus, an educational interpreter can avoid serving dual roles, because they cannot both interpret and participate in the IEP meeting. However, not all school districts will secure an outside interpreter so the educational interpreter can attend the IEP meeting. If the school district requires the interpreter to interpret the IEP meeting rather than attend, they should make sure that any notes or observations that they have are given to another member of the IEP Team before the meeting. Even if the educational interpreter is not invited to attend and contribute to the IEP meeting, they are still a member of the child's IEP Team.

IEP meetings must occur at least annually, though parents may request an IEP meeting or school personnel may call an IEP meeting at any time. Decisions about the child's education including goals, placement, and services must be determined by the IEP Team. It is illegal for team members to decide on any of these aspects without input from the IEP Team, a violation known as *predetermination of services*. The team must discuss the child's PLAAFP and, from that, determine the services necessary for the child to receive a FAPE. Then the placement decision should be made based on where the child can receive the services they need. Team members can bring recommendations to IEP meetings based on data collected, but no decisions can be made without approval from the IEP Team (which must include parents, an administrator, teachers, and someone qualified to interpret assessment data).

IEP meetings typically proceed in a prescribed manner: introductions, rights and safeguards, student strengths and concerns, transition needs (if applicable), academic performance and goals, services, placement, and prior written notice (PWN). After the team members introduce themselves and their roles, the parents are offered a copy of their rights and safeguards. This is part of the procedural requirements of the IEP. Following this, the team discusses the strengths and areas of concern for the child, with input from the parents. If the child is in high school, there is usually a discussion of the child's transition needs (i.e., what their goals are post-high school and what supports they may need to attain those goals). The team then reviews the child's current academic performance, identifies areas where they have an educational need, and reviews the goals they have established to support the child in closing their academic gaps. This is followed by identifying services the child needs to receive a FAPE, and discussion of the least restrictive environment (LRE) where the child can receive a FAPE. During the IEP meeting, one team member is tasked with taking notes, usually an administrator or IEP coordinator. These notes include decisions agreed upon by the team, which are then used to generate a PWN. The PWN is another one of the procedural requirements of the IEP.

There is a great deal of controversy between the Deaf community and the broader education community about how to interpret LRE for Deaf children. In broader SPED terms, mainstream placement with non-disabled peers is considered the LRE. As language and communication are often barriers for Deaf students interacting with their hearing peers, many Deaf people believe that mainstream placements are the most restrictive (Conference of Educational Administrators of Schools and Programs for the Deaf, Inc., 2019; National Association of the Deaf, 2002).

Placements

As mentioned, there are different types of educational placements available to Deaf children. The bedrock of SPED in the United States is the IDEA law. One of the founding principles of IDEA is *inclusion*, as in disabled and non-disabled students being educated together. Therefore, the goal of IDEA is to reduce the amount of time that students in SPED are pulled from the general education classroom in order to work in a self-contained, resource, or other specialized setting.

However, for Deaf students, this practice leads to isolation and exclusion because of language or communication barriers between Deaf students and their hearing peers (Oliva & Risser Lytle, 2014; Ramsey, 1997; Reed, Antia, & Kreimeyer, 2008; Nunes, Pretzlik, & Olsson, 2001; Shaver, Marschark, Newman, & Marder, 2014; Winston, 2004). Therefore, for many Deaf students, a state school for the Deaf is the most inclusive, and least restrictive environment. However, because most educators operate from a SPED, hearing lens, their interpretation of the LRE is "integration into mainstream programming." Thus, students with disabilities who do not require academic support will spend all of their time mainstreamed in general education and may receive consultation services from service providers as needed.

Some students need direct services to support their learning. In such cases, every attempt is made to provide those supports in the general education classroom through what is called *push-in* services (Rabinsky, 2013). For example, a reading specialist may come into a general education classroom and provide direct support to a student during English Language Arts instruction. The opposite of push-in services are *pull-out* services, where the student leaves the general education classroom to go to a separate room.

Resource Room

Another type of placement is the resource room. This is where students can go during certain times of the day for SPED- or Deaf Ed-related services. This may include pull-out time for speech language pathology, audiology, instruction from a teacher of the Deaf, and specially designed instruction with a SPED teacher. The teacher in charge of a resource room is usually a SPED teacher, and students using the resource room typically spend the bulk of their day with the general education population. The most common resource room supports are in literacy and math instruction.

Self-Contained Classrooms

Another type of placement that is considered more restrictive is a self-contained classroom. Self-contained classrooms only serve students with disabilities, so they are considered more restrictive because of the lack of interaction with non-disabled peers.

The term self-contained is commonly used, but it has some negative connotations. Some schools have what are called *cluster sites*, where all of the students in a particular school district with the same disability are sent to the same building. In Deaf Ed, this practice is more common in larger school districts with more Deaf students and serves as a way of pooling resources as well as giving Deaf students social opportunities with their Deaf peers.

At cluster site schools, the resource room or self-contained classroom for Deaf students is run by a Teacher of the Deaf, and Deaf students have more opportunities for *direct instruction* (when a student is learning directly from their teacher and not through an interpreter). IDEA requires the educational team to consider the opportunities that a Deaf child has for direct communication (but not direct instruction) with their teachers and peers (United States Department of Education, Office for Civil Rights, 1992; United States Department of Education, Office of Special Education Programs, 2010; 2011).

DC: I was consulting with a school district on the language needs of a Deaf student. In the student's IEP, the team listed "hugs," "smiles," and "waves" as the "opportunities for direct communication" the Deaf student had with their peers. People's pets have more opportunities for direct communication than that Deaf student.

Separate Schools

The "most restrictive" setting is a separate school, such as a state residential school for the Deaf. At a residential school for the Deaf, students have an opportunity for direct instruction from their teachers all day long, and direct interactions with their peers all day long. Ironically, this may be considered to be the LRE for Deaf students.

Unfortunately, in many states, schools for the Deaf have closed or shrunk over the decades since IDEA became law. State schools for the Deaf are often seen as a last-resort placement for Deaf students once they have fallen behind in general education. Despite years of research on Deaf mental health, language deprivation, and social emotional needs saying otherwise, the practice of mainstreaming Deaf students first is the most prevalent in the United States. Therefore, there is a high demand for educational interpreters.

Educational Interpreters and Placements

Educational interpreter responsibilities look different depending on the type of placement, as well as the student's age, language fluency, maturity, understanding of interpreter role and function, and academic level (Winston, 2015). The setting that looks most like stereotypical community interpreting is at the secondary level with a student who is linguistically and academically on par with their peers. These students are preparing to transition into the world, and function relatively independently in the school setting, using their interpreter services primarily just for access to the classroom.

However, educational interpreters need to be prepared to work with students in all settings. One facet of working in resource or self-contained settings is that educational interpreters are often tasked with more responsibilities akin to those of a paraprofessional, which include monitoring student behavior, preparing support materials, toileting, and other personal hygiene. It is important to be aware of how much of your time is spent doing paraprofessional-type duties for the student with whom you are working. If you are functioning more like a paraprofessional than an interpreter, you would want to take this information back to the IEP Team. This is particularly relevant for students with severe cognitive disabilities who may or may not have a great deal of expressive or receptive language. They may be better served by a paraprofessional who is fluent in ASL than by an educational interpreter. However, the shortage of ASL-fluent paraprofessionals often results in school districts, particularly small ones with few resources, combining the responsibilities of multiple professionals into one job description.

It is a critical part of ethical practice that educational interpreters understand the job description they are being hired with, and that they understand something of the setting and needs of the student for whom they are hired (Antia & Kreimeyer, 2001; Fitzmaurice, 2021; Kurz & Metzger, 2021). This is especially true for small school districts where there may be only one educational interpreter in the school district to serve a single Deaf student for the duration of that student's education (Fitzmaurice, 2017; Yarger, 2001).

If an educational interpreter is filling multiple roles on a regular basis, the educational placement is likely not an appropriate fit for the Deaf child to receive a FAPE. Furthermore, if an educational interpreter continues to fill multiple roles without bringing it to the attention of the IEP Team and school administration, there will never be a reason for the team to question the appropriateness of the placement.

Collaboration

For Deaf students on an IEP, special factors will include communication needs, linguistic needs, hearing level, academic level, and opportunities for direct communication with peers. Educational interpreters can provide valuable insight to the IEP Team about the child's use of language in different environments. The educational interpreter is the only Related Service Provider who spends the entire school day with the Deaf child. Even a child who is in a classroom with a teacher of the Deaf all day will still go out for special classes, such as art or physical education (PE). Therefore, the educational interpreter is the only Related Service Provider who sees the child in all settings of their school day (Fitzmaurice, 2021). As a member of the student's IEP Team, the interpreter will share information about interpreted interactions in a way that they would not for an adult Deaf person. This is one of the key differences between interpreting in educational settings and interpreting in community settings. Educational interpreters must still maintain confidentiality, but that does not include confidentiality from members of the IEP Team. This topic is discussed in more depth later in this volume under ethical decision-making.

The educational interpreter should inform the IEP Team about what language the child is using, how the child is using that language, how they are attending to the interpreter in classes, how the student communicates with their teachers and peers, and areas where the educational interpreter has noted the student is having difficulty with language. These are all points of data to which the educational interpreter has access in their daily work with students. Interpreters may collect data on and/or have goals around the student's use of their interpreting services. For example, there may be certain classes, environments, or situations where the interpreter notices the student is looking at them more frequently or for more sustained periods. This may be just a point of data for the IEP Team, or it may be connected to a goal around the student learning to appropriately attend to their interpreter. For students who use both ASL and spoken English, they may attend more to the person speaking than to their interpreter signing. This may give rise to the educational team considering pulling the interpreter services. In such instances, observations from the educational interpreter about how and when the student is accessing their services may prove invaluable to the team's decision-making process.

DC: I once worked with an educational interpreter who worked with a senior in high school. The team was discussing transition planning, and whether or not the Deaf student would need an interpreter in college. Members of the IEP Team who had done classroom observations did not see the student looking at the interpreter at all. The interpreter tracked how often the student glanced at them during classes over the course of a week and charted these glances into a graph. The graph showed that when teachers covered new material in a couple of the more challenging classes, and when the student had been working late the night before, there were substantially more glances at the interpreter. This data helped show the value of interpreter services for this student.

Where Do Educational Interpreters Fit in?

The specific work of educational interpreters is addressed in chapter seven; however, we believe it is important to share the perceptions of educational interpreters by different members of the team. In brief, we know educational interpreters are part of the IEP Team and are considered professional Related Service Providers. However, we also know district and school administrators (think principals and vice-principals) and most teachers view the role of an educational interpreter as subordinate to teachers (Fitzmaurice, 2021). Administrators generally perceive the teacher of the Deaf as responsible for the education of Deaf children, whereas both general education teachers and teachers of the Deaf view the educational interpreter as being responsible for the education of Deaf students. In fact, the vast majority of administrators perceive the work of educational interpreters as adhering to a conduit-like metaphor (see chapter six) (Fitzmaurice, 2021).

Although we have an extremely important role for providing access to Deaf students, there is still much systemic confusion on what educational interpreters are, and how they fit into the education system.

Guiding Documents and Resources

There are a few documents that any educational interpreter should be aware of. The first one is the IDEA law (Individuals with Disabilities Education Act, 2004). This is the law that governs SPED. It is critical for interpreters to understand what their requirements and responsibilities are pursuant to IDEA law for Related Service Providers.

Likewise, educational interpreters should be familiar with the ADA (Americans with Disabilities Act, 1990). Under the ADA, the "effective communication" clause is intended to ensure a Deaf person can effectively communicate with, receive, and convey information. The defining factors related to communicating effectively are rooted in the nature, length, complexity, and context of the communication. In addition, the person's normal preferred method of communication must be considered (United States Department of Justice, Civil Rights Division, n.d.).

Another guidance document that every educational interpreter should be familiar with is "the purple book"—*Optimizing Outcomes for Students who are Deaf or Hard of Hearing: Educational Service Guidelines* (National Association of State Directors of Special Education, 2019). The purple book has all of the most recent guidance, descriptions, and information from the Directors of SPED about Deaf Ed. As discussed above, SPED and Deaf Ed are not the same thing. However, it is not uncommon for people who work in SPED to be over those who work in Deaf Ed. Therefore, it is an important document because it will help educational interpreters understand the SPED perception of Deaf Ed. This book is also excellent for helping educational interpreters to explain how their role and function may differ from the role and function of other service providers within Deaf Ed. It is not uncommon for people in general education (teachers and administrators) to not quite understand the differences between an educational interpreter, a teacher of the Deaf, and a paraprofessional.

Interpreters should also be aware of the NAIE *Professional Guidelines for Interpreting in Educational Settings* (National Association of Interpreters in Education, 2019). The guidelines contain information about the recommended credentials, job title, job description, duties, and responsibilities of an educational interpreter. When school districts have not previously worked with educational interpreters, they likely do not know how to develop an appropriate job description or expectations for educational interpreters. These documents can provide support to educational interpreters working to make changes to such within their districts.

Ethical guidance documents are another important resource for educational interpreters. These include the NAIE *Educational Interpreter Code of Ethics* (National Association of Interpreters in Education, 2021) as well as the Registry of Interpreters for the Deaf (RID) *Code of Professional Conduct* (RIDCPC) (National Association of the Deaf & Registry of Interpreters for the Deaf, 2005). These documents are discussed in detail in chapter six and provide some guiding tenets to help interpreters make informed ethical decisions, as well as to engage in *reflective practice*.

It may also be helpful to be aware of approaches to behavior management for students, though the responsibility for behavior management should not fall on an educational interpreter. However, it is important for interpreters to understand the principles of the Positive Behavior Intervention System (PBIS) as one of the most common approaches for behavior management in schools. For example, Missouri has information publicly available about the PBIS system (Missouri Schoolwide Positive Behavior Support, n.d.). This is beneficial for educational interpreters to have as a reference. There are also PBIS modules that are available through Vanderbilt University and are helpful for foundational information in SPED.

Lastly, in addition to these national documents, there may be a state handbook for educational interpreters. Educational interpreters should check and see if this is something that their SDE has prepared.

Summary

This chapter examined the influence of Public Law 94–142 (now IDEA) on Deaf education, and described how the education system is structured across federal, state, and local levels. We detailed Individualized Education Programs (IEPs) and 504 Plans and described a variety of educational placements for Deaf students. Those can include mainstreaming, resource rooms, self-contained classrooms, and completely separate schools.

We note educational interpreters play a vital role in these settings, adapting their approach based on the placement. At the secondary level, educational interpreters primarily provide communication access for independent students. However, in resource or self-contained settings, educational interpreters may take on paraprofessional duties like behavior monitoring and personal care, especially when working with students with cognitive disabilities. If an educational interpreter's role leans heavily toward paraprofessional tasks, it may indicate an inappropriate placement for the Deaf child.

We also shared some guiding documents that educational interpreters should be familiar with including IDEA, ADA provisions on effective communication, and NAIE's professional guidelines and code of ethics. These documents help define an educational interpreter's role and ensure ethical practice. Understanding behavior intervention systems can also be beneficial in behavior management, though this should not primarily be the interpreter's responsibility.

Thought Questions

1. What is the educational interpreter's responsibility on the IEP Team? How does the status of Related Service Provider differ from the work of community interpreting?
2. Educational interpreters need to know about goals, structures, and levels of language in discourse. Why is this important?
3. Do you believe mainstream classrooms are the least restrictive environment for Deaf students? Why or why not?

References

Alawajee, O. (2022). Exploring the sign language proficiency of university undergraduate students in a preservices preparation program for teachers of deaf students. *Higher Education Pedagogies*, 7(1), 65–87. doi:10.1080/23752696.2022.2092882.

Americans with Disabilities Act of 1990, 42 U.S.C. §§ 12101–12213 (2018).

Antia, S. D., & Kreimeyer, K. H. (2001). The role of interpreters in inclusive classrooms. *American Annals of the Deaf*, 146(4), 355–365.

Beal-Alvarez, J. S., & Scheetz, N. A. (2015). Preservice teacher and interpreter American Sign Language abilities: Self-evaluations and evaluations of deaf students' narrative renditions. *American Annals of the Deaf*, 160(3), 316–333.

Board of Education of the Hendrick Hudson Central School District v. Rowley, 458 U.S. 176 (1982).

Colorado Department of Education. (2014). *Expanded core curriculum for students who are deaf or hard of hearing: A guide for families and professionals*. Colorado Springs: Colorado School for the Deaf and the Blind.

Conference of Educational Administrators of Schools and Programs for the Deaf, Inc. (2019). What constitutes the least restrictive environment for a deaf or hard of hearing student?Mount Rainier, MD: CEASD. https://www.ceasd.org/wp-content/uploads/2019/10/What-Constitutes-the-Least-Restrictive-Environment-for-a-Deaf-or-Hard-of-Hearing-Student.pdf.

Council for Exceptional Children. (n.d.). Specially designed instruction. Retrieved April 28, 2025, from https://exceptionalchildren.org/topics/specially-designed-instruction.

Educational Audiology Association. (2019). Educational audiology scope of practice. https://edaud.org/pdf/scope-of-practice.pdf.

Endrew F. v. Douglas County School District Re-1, 580 U.S. 386 (2017).

Fitzmaurice, S. (2017). Unregulated autonomy: Uncredentialed educational interpreters in rural schools. *American Annals of the Deaf*, 162(3), 253–264.

Fitzmaurice, S. B. (2021). *The role of the educational interpreter: Perceptions of administrators and teachers*. Washington, DC: Gallaudet University Press.

Guardino, C. (2015). Evaluating teachers' preparedness to work with students who are Deaf and hard of hearing with disabilities. *American Annals of the Deaf*, 160(4), 415–426.

Individuals with Disabilities Education Act, 20 U.S.C. §§ 1400–1482 (2004).

Iowa Department of Education. (2019). *The expanded core curriculum for students who are Deaf or hard of hearing*. Des Moines: Iowa Department of Education. https://educate.iowa.gov/media/6522/download?inline=.

Knoors, H., & Marschark, M. (2014). *Teaching deaf learners: Psychological and developmental foundations*. New York: Oxford University Press.

Kurz, K. B., & Metzger, M. (2021). Signed language interpreters in education: Perspectives on their role in deaf and hard of hearing students' educational placement. In E. A. Winston & S. B. Fitzmaurice (Eds.), *Advances in educational interpreting* (pp. 352–370). Washington, DC: Gallaudet University Press.

Lane, H. (1992). *The mask of benevolence: Disabling the Deaf community*. New York: Knopf.

Lane, H. (1999). *The mask of benevolence: Disabling the deaf community*. San Diego, CA: DawnSignPress.

LaPlante, M. (2023, August 24). UnDisciplined: 'It's one of the most lonely feelings': The realities of mainstream schooling for deaf children. Upr.org. https://www.upr.org/show/undisciplined/2023-08-24/undisciplined-its-one-of-the-most-lonely-feelings-the-realities-of-mainstream-schooling-for-deaf-children.

Luckner, J. L., & Ayantoye, C. (2013). Itinerant teachers of students who are deaf or hard of hearing: Practices and preparation. *Journal of Deaf Studies and Deaf Education*, 18(3), 409–423.

Marschark, M., & Hauser, P. C. (2012). *How deaf children learn: What parents and teachers need to know*. New York: Oxford University Press.

Missouri Schoolwide Positive Behavior Support. (n.d.). *Missouri schoolwide positive behavior support*. Retrieved April 30, 2025, from https://pbismissouri.org/.

National Association of Interpreters in Education. (2019). Professional guidelines for interpreting in educational settings (1st ed.). Retrieved April 30, 2025, from https://naiedu.org/guidelines/.

National Association of Interpreters in Education. (2021). Educational interpreter code of ethics. Retrieved April 30, 2025, from https://naiedu.org/codeofethics/.

National Association of State Directors of Special Education. (2019). *Optimizing outcomes for students who are Deaf or hard of hearing: Educational service guidelines*. Alexandria, VA: National Association of State Directors of Special Education.

National Association of the Deaf. (2002). Position statement on inclusion. Silver Spring, MD: National Association of the Deaf. https://www.nad.org/about-us/position-statements/position-statement-on-inclusion/.

National Association of the Deaf. (n.d.). Position statement: Educating PreK–12 deaf and hard of hearing students during the COVID-19 outbreak. Silver Spring, MD: National Association of the Deaf. https://www.nad.org/position-statement-educating-prek-12-deaf-and-hard-of-hearing-students-during-the-covid-19-outbreak/.

National Association of the Deaf & Registry of Interpreters for the Deaf. (2005). Code of professional conduct. Retrieved April 30, 2025, from https://rid.org/programs/ethics/code-of-professional-conduct/.

National Deaf Center on Postsecondary Outcomes. (2018). Deaf students in public schools. Austin, TX: National Deaf Center on Postsecondary Outcomes.

Nunes, T., Pretzlik, U., & Olsson, J. (2001). Deaf children's social relationships in mainstream schools. *Journal of Deaf Education International*, 3(3), 123–136.

Oliva, G. A., & Risser Lytle, L. (2014). *Turning the tide: Making life better for deaf and hard of hearing schoolchildren*. Washington, DC: Gallaudet University Press.

Perez v. Sturgis Public Schools, 598 U.S. 142 (2023).

Rabinsky, R. J. (2013). Itinerant deaf educator and general educator perceptions of the D/HH push-in model. *American Annals of the Deaf*, 158(1), 50–62.

Ramsey, C. (1997). *Deaf children in public schools: Placement, context, and consequences*. Washington, DC: Gallaudet University Press.

Reed, S., Antia, S. D., & Kreimeyer, K. H. (2008). Academic status of deaf and hard-of-hearing students in public schools: Student, home, and service facilitators and detractors. *Journal of Deaf Studies and Deaf Education*, 13(4), 485–502.

Rehabilitation Act of 1973, 29 U.S.C. §§ 701–796l (2018).

Shaver, D. M., Marschark, M., Newman, L., & Marder, C. (2014). Who is where? Characteristics of deaf and hard-of-hearing students in regular and special schools. *Journal of Deaf Studies and Deaf Education, 19*(2), 203–219.

Supporting Success for Children with Hearing Loss. (2024, March). Addressing the shortage of deaf and hard of hearing teachers. https://successforkidswithhearingloss.com/wp-content/uploads/2024/03/Addressing-the-Shortage-of-Deaf-and-Hard-of-Hearing.pdf.

Swanepoel, D. W., & Störbeck, C. (2022). Exploring the sign language proficiency of university undergraduate preservice teachers of deaf students. *Deafness & Education International*, 24(3), 181–194.

United States Department of Education, Office for Civil Rights. (1992). Deaf students education services. https://www2.ed.gov/about/offices/list/ocr/docs/hq9806.html.

United States Department of Education, Office of Special Education Programs. (2010). Policy letter to Conference of Educational Administrators of Schools and Programs for the Deaf, Inc. https://sites.ed.gov/idea/idea-files/policy-letter-august-23-2010-to-conference-of-educational-administrators-of-schools-and-programs-for-the-deaf-inc-president-edward-h-bosso-jr/.

United States Department of Education, Office of Special Education Programs. (2011). Policy letter to Conference of Educational Administrators of Schools and Programs for the Deaf, Inc. https://sites.ed.gov/idea/files/idea/policy/speced/guid/idea/letters/2011-3/stern093011lre3q2011.pdf.

United States Department of Justice, Civil Rights Division. (n.d.). ADA requirements: Effective communication. https://www.ada.gov/resources/effective-communication/.

Waddy-Smith, B., & Wilson, M. (2003). *See the sound: Visual phonics*. See the Sound/Visual Phonics, Inc.

Winston, E. A. (2004). Interpretability and accessibility of mainstream classrooms. In E. A. Winston (Ed.), *Educational interpreting: How it can succeed* (pp. 132–167). Washington, DC: Gallaudet University Press.

Winston, E. A. (2015). Educational interpreting. Setting. Signed language interpreting. In F. Pöchhacker (Ed.), *Routledge encyclopedia of interpreting studies* (pp. 130–135). New York, NY: Routledge.

Yarger, C. C. (2001). Educational interpreting: Understanding the rural experience. *American Annals of the Deaf*, 146(1), 16–30.

4 The Curriculum and Academic Content Areas

Educational Discourse

The work interpreters do is fundamentally rooted in discourse analysis (Roy, 2000). They take an incoming discourse in one language and interpret it into discourse in another language. This goes beyond just knowing the word or sign for a concept. American Sign Language (ASL) and English are two different languages. They have different grammatical structure and vocabulary, and both are shaped by different cultural and pragmatic norms.

Interpreters must process information as they work, analyzing it for the goal, main ideas, and key details and vocabulary (Cates, 2021; Metzger, 1995a). In educational settings, discourse is guided by the curriculum, which is covered later in this chapter. Here, we discuss interpreter processing at each level of discourse.

Goal-Driven Processing

Information processing is either top-down or bottom-up. Applied to interpreting, top-down processing is when the goal and structure of the discourse drive the choices an interpreter makes in how they structure and deliver their interpretation. Bottom-up processing is when the words or signs in the source message drive the choices an interpreter makes in how they structure and deliver their interpretation. If an interpreter does not understand the goal of a discourse, it is difficult to achieve dynamic equivalence. Students of interpreting are often tempted to think of interpreting as finding single word and sign equivalents. "I don't know the sign(s) for that" is a common refrain. This is the morphological level of language, and it is a hallmark of bottom-up processing.

Interpreting is so much more than just signing a series of signs or speaking a series of words. All of it starts with the goal of the discourse. The reason somebody is talking drives the work that the interpreter is doing. The goal influences message management features such as omissions, compressions, and expansions. Some aspects of ASL, such as fingerspelling, take substantially more time to produce than their English equivalents. Conversely, some aspects of

DOI: 10.4324/9781003423058-4

ASL, such as directional verbs, take substantially less time to produce than their English equivalents, especially once spatial referents have been established. If interpreters understand why somebody is talking, they can more efficiently manage their use of discourse space, which in turn allows more time for them to fingerspell or use other ASL discourse features that may take more time to produce.

For example, if a teacher is teaching on photosynthesis and their goal is for students to understand the ingredients in photosynthesis, the interpreter may structure their interpretation as a list, with each ingredient of photosynthesis being an item in that list. However, if the teacher's goal is for students to understand the reactants and products of photosynthesis, the interpreter may structure their interpretation as a cause/effect with reactants on one side of their signing space and products on the other side of their signing space. Those two interpretations would be driven by top-down processing. If the interpreter was relying on bottom-up processing, their representation of the material would look very similar—they would sign about SUNLIGHT, WATER, CHLOROPHYLL, CARBON DIOXIDE, SUGAR, and OXYGEN—but the differing goals of knowing the ingredients of photosynthesis versus the reactants and products in the equation of photosynthesis would not be transparent. Top-down processing ensures the interpreter is keeping the goal of the discourse at the center of their interpretation to achieve dynamic equivalence.

Top-down processing guides how interpreters structure information in the target language. In an educational setting, the interpreter must understand the teacher's goals because they are driven by curriculum, which is the overarching sequence of the student's education. If an interpreter understands the sequence of the curriculum, and they understand the goal of a teacher's lesson, then they can produce an interpretation that reflects the scaffolded nature of the material.

Language Structure

There are multiple levels of language structure, and each level gives a different challenge to sign language interpreters in their work. The lowest level is phonological structure, which deals with the individual sounds of words and parameters of signs (i.e., handshape, location, movement, palm orientation). Aside from knowing the correct pronunciation of a word or sign, this level presents challenges to educational interpreters most often during early literacy instruction. Literacy instruction usually begins with phonological awareness in English. Signed languages have phonological structure, but there is no connection between sign phonology and print the way there is with spoken language phonology and print for languages with alphabetic writing systems like English. ASL rhymes and handshape games are excellent resources for interpreters working with young Deaf children, as research has shown a link between ASL phonological awareness and English print literacy.

DC: I was doing an observation once of a Deaf first grader and their interpreter during phonics. The lesson was on phoneme substitution (i.e., "sink," replace /s/ with /p/ and you get "pink"). The student is bilingual in ASL and English and uses cochlear implants. However, the student had some early language deprivation, so they do not know as many words for familiar concepts as their classmates. The interpreter was trying to give the student exposure to the print word, sound pattern, visual phonics gestural cue, visual phonics print cue, ASL sign, spelling, and definition of the word. The Deaf student's peers only had to worry about the print word, sound pattern, and spelling. The Deaf student and their interpreter were doing twice as much work as everyone else.

The next level of language structure is morphological. This level deals with the smallest units of language that have meaning. In English, morphological structure is often highlighted during English language arts lessons on verb tense. For example, the English word endings -ing and -ed have the respective meanings of continuous or past time when added to the ends of verbs. Educational interpreters will also see morphology frequently in lessons on word roots and affixes, which are common in subjects with more advanced or specialized vocabulary. This level of discourse presents challenges to educational interpreters because morphology in ASL is rarely expressed through sequential affixation (i.e., go + ing is "going"). Instead, one or more parameters of the sign change such that affixation is simultaneous. For example, continuous time in ASL is expressed with a circular movement. Pluralization is expressed with a repeated or sweeping movement. Handshapes for time signs can change to incorporate number (e.g., ONE-MONTH, TWO-MONTH, THREE-MONTH). One sequential affix ASL does have is PERSON (agent), which is similar in function to the English affix -er. These affixes derive nouns from verbs (e.g., law/lawyer, LAW/LAW-PERSON). Educational interpreters should study word roots and be prepared to break words down visually to show their component meanings while interpreting.

The next level of language structure is syntactic. This level deals with the way in which words are combined to form phrases and sentences. One way in which ASL and English syntax differ substantially is in how *figure* and *ground* are established. "Figure" is the object of interest, and "ground" is the environment around the figure. For example, assume that the figure in the following sentence is "house." In English, you could have a sentence such as, "There is a house on the hill in the middle of a corn field surrounded by a low wooden fence." In ASL, you would establish the CORN FIELD first, then the FENCE, then the HILL, then the HOUSE. You establish the ground first, and then the figure. Such differences in sentence structure pose a challenge to interpreters during story time and to Deaf students during writing time in English classes. One popular bilingual instruction method is to sign sentences twice while reading—once with sign equivalents for each word following English word order and fingerspelling elements of English grammar (i.e., the, is, an), and then again interpreted into grammatically accurate ASL. Educational interpreters can adopt this practice, modeling both ways of reading sentences "aloud" in ASL to form connections between English and ASL sentence structures.

The highest level of language structure is the discourse level. This level includes the goal, structure, and cohesive features of the entire discourse. Every discourse has a purpose. For example, right now, you are reading this textbook, and the purpose of this discourse is to teach you the principles of ASL-English educational interpreting. Therefore, this textbook is written in such a way that you will be able to learn about ASL-English educational interpreting (we hope).

Goals of Discourse

There are six fundamental goals of discourse. In other words, there are six basic reasons people communicate with one another. These purposes are narrative, explanatory, argumentative, hortatory, procedural, and conversational (Martin & Rose, 2008; Paltridge, 2013).

Narrative discourse tries to tell a story. An example of a narrative discourse would be story time in an elementary school when the teacher is reading to children to expose them to a story. When interpreting narrative discourse, educational interpreters will use extensive role shift, depiction, and facial expression to convey characters and their actions.

Explanatory discourse should explain why or how something happens or has occurred, but does not simply mean that somebody is explaining something. An explanatory discourse will be structured in such a way that every major idea from that structure supports an explanation of why or how something specific has happened. The goal of teacher discourse is often explanatory. This textbook is an example of an explanatory discourse. It is structured such that everything in this book is explaining some of why educational interpreting is what it is, or how to function as an educational interpreter. There is some narrative in this book, as both authors have shared some of their personal experiences in order to help you understand what the world of educational interpreting looks like. However, these narratives are not there simply to tell stories about the interpreting profession. They are included to show you how the information in this textbook applies to the real work of educational interpreting. When interpreting explanatory discourse, educational interpreters will structure their interpretation around the why or how.

An argumentative discourse tries to prove something. One hallmark of argumentative discourse is that there are two sides, such as in a political debate. Each side is trying to argue a point against the other side. This is in contrast with hortatory discourse, wherein there are no sides. In hortatory discourse, the goal is to persuade somebody to think, feel, or believe something. Hortatory discourse usually has one of three types of appeals: ethos, pathos, or logos. Ethos is an argument that appeals to your sense of what is credible, pathos is an argument that appeals to your emotions, and logos is an argument that appeals to your sense of logic. Whereas a political debate is an example of argumentative discourse, someone trying to convince you to become a registered voter is an example of a hortatory discourse. In educational settings, argumentative and hortatory discourses occur most frequently in speech and debate courses, as well as English classes when students must write argumentative or persuasive essays. When interpreting argumentative discourse, educational interpreters will have a clear set-up in space where the arguments from each side are kept separate in right-space and left-space. When interpreting hortatory discourse, educational interpreters will identify the type of appeal (ethos, pathos, logos) and will use posture and affect to highlight it.

In a procedural discourse, the goal is to get you to follow or understand a process. Procedural discourse usually involves a series of steps that result in a product. Examples of procedural discourses include science labs, recipes in cooking classes, and instructions for projects in art classes. When interpreting procedural discourse, educational interpreters will organize their interpretation in a temporal structure with clear time markers showing the order of the steps in the process.

In conversational discourse, the goal is usually relational. In educational settings, teachers sometimes use conversational-style discourse to build rapport with students. Students use conversational discourse with one another to play, make friends, and flirt. Interpreters face challenges with conversational discourse when interpreting peer-to-peer interactions. It can be awkward for students to have conversations with their friends through an interpreter who is an adult and who may lack the same demographics as the student group (gender, age, race, culture, etc.) (Kurz & Langer, 2004; Langer & Schick, 2004; Oliva & Risser Lytle, 2014). When interpreting for teachers using a conversational style, educational interpreters will change their register to indicate the teacher's purpose.

DC: One of my male-presenting colleagues tells an amusing but bittersweet story about interpreting for a pre-teen Deaf girl who wanted to ask her friends about their periods. Needless to say, the girls did not say much!

Information Structure

Just as there are six primary goals of discourse, so there are six structural relationships that ideas can have within a discourse. These relationships are coordinated, causal, sequential, cyclical, couched, and comparative (Gee, 2011; Martin & Rose, 2008; Van Dijk & Kintsch, 1983). Coordinated ideas are ideas that relate to one another but have no particular order, and they are usually presented as lists. Examples of common lists in educational settings include lists of supplies needed for a project, lists of characters in a story, and lists of vocabulary words at the start of a new unit. Causal ideas are ideas that have a cause/effect relationship to one another, such as the causes of wars that we learn about in history classes. Sequential ideas are ideas that have a temporal ordering; that is, the order in which they occur matters. For example, the steps of an experiment in science class will be ordered sequentially. Cyclical ideas are ideas that have a temporal ordering that repeats. Cyclical ideas may have defined start and end points, such as mitosis or the life cycle, or they may have no definitive beginning or ending, such as the water cycle. Couched, or hierarchical, ideas are larger wholes made up of smaller parts. Examples of these include family trees, organ systems, and sentence diagrams. Comparative ideas are ideas that are compared or contrasted with one another for the purpose of highlighting similarities or differences between them. For example, students may be asked to compare two narrative accounts in English class, or to contrast types of government in social studies.

An easy way to see an illustration of these relationships is to look at graphic organizers (Zaini, Mokhtar, & Nawawi, 2010). The purpose of graphic organizers is to lay out information from a discourse in a spatial way that shows the relationships between ideas. They are a great tool for interpreters to use to analyze the main ideas and structure of texts. A bonus is that the spatial layout of a graphic organizer can translate directly into the interpreter's sign space when working into ASL to help keep the discourse organized and lend cohesion to the interpreted product.

Cohesion and Coherence

There are two separate but related principles that drive the work an interpreter does. The first principle is the principle of cohesion. Cohesion is a property of a discourse. A discourse that is cohesive has a logical flow, and all of the internal elements are connected. There are two different ways in which discourse is cohesive. The first is through relationships between words within a discourse that make it obvious that the discourse is all about one singular point or topic. This is called lexical cohesion. The other way to generate cohesion is with grammatical structure. This is called grammatical cohesion.

Lexical cohesion connects a discourse through the relationships that words within the discourse have with one another. These relationships might be words with a similar meaning (synonyms), words that have opposite meanings (antonyms), words that typically occur together such as paper/plastic and peanut butter/jelly (collocation), and use of repetition. In another part of this book, we address the principles of fingerspelling, and its importance in educational settings. We talk about techniques called sandwiching and chaining. These techniques make fingerspelling cohesive with the rest of the signed discourse through repetition and synonymy. Later in this volume, we address some features of ASL discourse that have previously been termed "expansion techniques." These features of ASL discourse lend cohesion to a signed message through both lexical and grammatical means.

Grammatical cohesion is when a text's grammatical structure helps all pieces of the text to be related to one another appropriately. This means that when a new referent is introduced into a discourse, the speaker or signer makes it clear what this referent is. This may be just a name if everyone will likely understand what the referent is, or this may be a descriptor of who or what the referent is. Grammatical cohesion also requires that anytime a pronoun is used, there is a clear antecedent. If you are not familiar with those terms, a pronoun is a word that stands in place of a noun, and an antecedent is the noun being referenced by the pronoun. If it is not clear within a discourse what a pronoun is referring to, then that discourse lacks cohesion. Another example of grammatical cohesion is the use of a single word to substitute for an entire larger concept that was previously covered in the discourse. For example, in a contract, the opening clause usually clarifies who the parties in the contract are and then indicates a specific word that will refer to each party. For the rest of the contract, only those single words are used rather than the entirety of all entities' names. This is a feature of grammatical cohesion called substitution. Another property of grammatical cohesion is ellipsis. In ellipsis, an entire phrase can be omitted once it has been stated and is then implicitly understood in context. Consider this sentence: An interpreter may enjoy working with one student but may dislike working with another. In the phrase "but may dislike working with another," the phrases "an interpreter" and "student" are not repeated. However, when you read the sentence, you knew that the interpreter may dislike working with another student. That is the property of ellipsis. An interpreter always has the goal of creating a cohesive discourse in the target language.

Grammatical cohesion in ASL is fundamentally spatial in nature. ASL has four broad uses of space: comparative, temporal, performative, and perspective (Emmorey & Falgier, 2004; Winston, 1991). Comparative space utilizes the space on the signer's left and right, and sometimes the space in front of their torso. Comparative space is used to separate one or more ideas and may not be specifically for comparing and contrasting information. Temporal space is organized in one of two ways: over the signer's shoulder with the past behind and the future ahead, or horizontally in front of the signer with the past to the left and the future to the right.

Performative space is utilized when the signer surrogates for a referent to show an action rather than talk about it, sometimes called *constructed action* (Kurz, Mullaney, & Occhino, 2019; Metzger, 1995b). Surrogation, or constructed action, is when a signer takes on the mannerisms of a referent and becomes that referent, such as licking the back of the hand and running it over the head to show the action of a cat. Perspective space is used to show how things look. Perspective space uses a great deal of depictive (classifier) constructions (Emmorey & Herzig, 2003).

DC: I will never forget the day I learned about the use of listing on the non-dominant hand as a grammatical cohesive device. One of my interpreting tests from my training program included a text with a teacher recalling their work with a student who had autism. One of this student's interests was coffee brands, and one of their ways of settling themselves was to hear a list of all of the coffee brands you would find in a grocery store. The student would come into class every day and say, "Tell me all the coffees." I literally signed TELL-ME ALL COFFEE. When my professor was grading my test, she suggested signing COFFEE BRAND CL:5 BLURT-INFORMATION. At that moment, something clicked, and I realized that I had to spatially restructure information in order to make it grammatically cohesive in ASL. In this source text, the English phrase "all the coffees" means a list of coffee brands. COFFEE-BRAND CL:5 BLURT-INFORMATION structurally means the same thing in ASL—a list of coffee brands. If it is clear in the discourse that a student and teacher are talking to one another, and the signer is role shifted into the student's space when signing "COFFEE BRAND CL:5 BLURT-INFORMATION," and the verb BLURT-INFORMATION is produced with the palm facing the signer, it conveys the same thing as the English "tell me all the coffees." That was the day I stopped just signing and started interpreting.

Other than cohesion, the second property that drives the work an interpreter does is coherence. Coherence means that a discourse makes sense to the intended recipients. A discourse that is not cohesive is likely also incoherent. However, a discourse can be cohesive but entirely incoherent to some audiences. If you attended an academic conference on a subject in which you are not well-versed, most sessions would be incoherent to you regardless of how cohesive the presenters are. In the Educational Interpreter Performance Assessment (EIPA) in Action series from Boys Town National Research Hospital, you will see examples of interpreters at different EIPA levels. You will see the lack of cohesion in the product of interpreters with lower EIPA scores. The result is a discourse that is incoherent to viewers, especially children who are still developing their academic language and reasoning skills. We deal with considerations for generating coherence in more detail in the section on Deaf students in this textbook.

Interpreting exams such as the EIPA test an interpreter's ability to generate a cohesive text, since coherence is a property of discourse between users of a language. Therefore, interpreter programs are focused on cohesion in interpreting. However, one cannot interpret for a child with language deprivation the same way one interprets for a native signer (Arpino, 2022; Caselli, Wyatte, & Henner, 2020). Strategies for differentiating interpreting are rarely taught beyond the selection of different sign systems or "transliterating" versus "interpreting."

There are features of ASL discourse that have been identified in interpreting literature as "expansion techniques" (Lawrence, 2003). However, these are not optional features of the language that interpreters can choose to or not to employ as they work. These are features of ASL discourse used to generate both cohesion and coherence between users of ASL. They are only "expansions" when viewed in contrast to English discourse features.

In educational settings, these features are particularly relevant because of the instructional nature of educational discourse (Bloome et al., 2022; Cazden, 2001) and because ASL does not have a large standardized technical vocabulary. Furthermore, educational interpreters must often fill gaps in Deaf students' funds of knowledge. These gaps exist because Deaf children do not have the same opportunities to acquire information incidentally the same way their hearing peers can. Therefore, it is critical that interpreters understand how to use these features of ASL to generate coherence for the students whom they serve, and to create cohesion between fingerspelled words and the context in which they occur.

Teacher Talk (Register)

If you have taken a linguistics class, you may have learned that there are five registers of language: intimate, informal (or casual), consultative, formal, and frozen (Joos, 1962; Halliday & Hasan, 1976). Educational settings primarily exist at a consultative register. Sometimes in education you will interpret in a formal or an informal register, but usually the register will be consultative.

When we talk about register and educational settings, we are not talking about these levels of register. We are talking about how teachers engage in their classrooms, and how students know what teachers mean by the way in which they talk (Bloome et al., 2022; Cazden, 2001; Nunan, 1991; Sharpe, 2008). One common framework for teacher instruction is called initiate, respond, and evaluate (IRE) (Sinclair & Coulthard, 1975). This is a common discursive structure that we see in classrooms. The teacher asks a question (initiate), a student answers the question (respond), and the teacher indicates if the answer was correct or not (evaluate). There are specific ways that teachers indicate through their speech whose turn it is to talk, and what type of information they are seeking. How teachers shift between open classroom dialogue, question/answer sessions, lecture, and individual support to students is what we mean by register in the classroom.

Anecdotally, it is common for Deaf people to grow up thinking that hearing people know everything. This is largely because educational interpreters often do not interpret the IRE structure appropriately. They leave out guesses from hearing students or corrections from the teacher that indicate the hearing students got something wrong. In contrast, Deaf students are often corrected more than they are praised. By leaving out these important aspects of classroom register, the interpreter prevents the Deaf student from seeing their hearing peers make mistakes. This may leave the Deaf student feeling like they are the only one who ever gets the wrong answer (Fitzmaurice, 2017; Kurz & Langer, 2004; Lawson, 2021; Smith, 2013; Winston, 2001). Accurate interpretation of teacher register reflects when it is time to participate in a classroom discussion, when a student is being asked a question directly, or when it is time to attend to the teacher without interruption.

Introduction to Curriculum

We have detailed Deaf students' individual placements and how placement shapes the Deaf student's access to curriculum. However, regardless of the student's placement, educational interpreters need to understand curriculum in order to effectively interpret. Curriculum is based on educational standards. You may have heard of "core standards" before. Core standards are a set of goal statements describing what children should be able to do in core academic areas (math, English language arts, social studies, science). Each state adopts core standards, which are often found on state or district websites segmented by subjects and grade levels. These standards are a critically important resource for educational interpreters because they help interpreters determine the levels of competency expected in each area for each grade as well as what specific subject matter they should expect to have to interpret at each grade level. The specific curriculum used to teach these standards varies by district, but every curriculum is designed to align with a set of core standards. The standards are a blueprint of what should be taught and when, allowing educational interpreters to use them for prep material.

In addition to a formal curriculum that school systems implement in their classes, there is also the unwritten or hidden curriculum in all schools. The hidden curriculum includes developing values, beliefs, norms, and culture—in other words, the incidental lessons that students learn subconsciously as they move through the school day. Such incidental lessons come from, for example, whom students see reflected in posters and announcements in school, the way classroom seating is organized, the way they are given feedback and correction from their teachers, etc. Many of the lessons learned in school are not necessarily linked to what students are explicitly taught in the classroom. For instance, consider how students learn about sharing, punctuality, respect for authority, respect for peers, making friends, flirting, turn taking, and social politeness. Students may not receive, for example, formal instruction that it is impolite to invite themselves to someone's party or to share publicly that someone has bad breath. Instead, students learn this as a result of interactions in school with classmates and other school personnel. This type of learning is indispensable to social advancement, and facilitating this type of learning as an educational interpreter can be one of the most challenging aspects of the job because this hidden curriculum is largely *implicit* in the way people talk rather than being stated explicitly in a way that interpreters can easily capture (Jackson, 1968; Apple & King, 1977; Alsubaie, 2015; McLeod, 2023; Notre Dame Learning, 2021). Therefore, Deaf students are often labeled as rude or weird, because they have not learned these implicit lessons, which in turn affects their ability to successfully socialize with their hearing peers.

We often read about educational interpreters providing access to education or access to the curriculum. The key word here is access, and in light of the hidden curriculum, we must consider if it is possible for one person to provide access to both the academic curriculum and the hidden curriculum. In truth, educational interpreters can only provide limited access to the classroom because there are so many layers happening simultaneously in any classroom. Educational interpreters will find it easier to focus on the written curriculum and follow along with most of what the teacher is saying explicitly. The written curriculum is complex enough for educational interpreters to navigate, and the nuances of the hidden curriculum mount a greater challenge, particularly when the Deaf student has limited language skills. For example, it is difficult to explain sharing to a Deaf preschool or kindergarten student who has minimal language skills because, to the Deaf student, it just looks like you are taking their toy away and giving it to someone else. Sharing is an abstract concept that must be explained using language, and it is part of the hidden curriculum. By way of another example, it is difficult to interpret hearing-centric turn-taking behaviors given the delay in the interpreting process, which means the Deaf student is often left out of class discussions and associated opportunities for teacher feedback. Furthermore, since it is easier for the educational interpreter to skip interpreting the hearing student's wrong answer in order to interpret clearly the corrected answer given by the teacher, the Deaf student misses out on the fact that other students make mistakes too. Without exposure to other students' wrong answers, Deaf students are left with the assumption that hearing people know everything. The knowledge that all students make mistakes is a hugely important part of the hidden curriculum.

Expanded Core Curriculum

There is a need for an expanded core curriculum above and beyond the general curriculum that is unique to the needs of Deaf students. For example, state standards are a required part of educational programming for all students. However, some students need to develop specialized skills to meet such standards, requiring *specially designed instruction*. Tackling this need, educators in Iowa designed the *Expanded Core Curriculum for Students Who Are Deaf or Hard of Hearing* (Iowa Department of Education, 2019, originally published in 2010). In this expanded curriculum, specific goals are laid out in a targeted sequence, similar to how state standards are organized around areas of core instruction. However, these expanded core standards go beyond math, English language arts, social studies, and science to address specific areas that uniquely affect Deaf students. The major areas of the expanded core curriculum are:

- Audiology
- Career Education
- Communication
- Family Education
- Functional Skills for Educational Success
- Self-Determination and Advocacy
- Social-Emotional Skills
- Technology

There is also an *Expanded Core Curriculum for Blind and Visually Impaired* students, so interpreters who are working with DeafBlind students should be aware of the standards within both documents (McDonough, Sticken, & Haack, 2006).

The state, and specific school, in which you ultimately work may use this expanded core curriculum. Even if they do not, it is helpful to know what those standards are and how mastery in each is indicated, because some areas of the hidden curriculum are captured in the expanded core curriculum. Educational interpreters can use the expanded core curriculum to help them think about aspects of the hidden curriculum they can and should make explicit while interpreting, especially in the areas of functional skills for educational success, self-determination and advocacy, and social-emotional skills.

Testing Considerations

Now that we have a better idea of what the curriculum means, how do we determine if the Deaf student has successfully completed the objectives in the curriculum?

Ultimately, the education system tends to focus on the tangible outcomes of the designed curriculum. Competencies in each component of the curriculum are typically identified in state standards with details of student performance at different grade levels (i.e., what the student should know and what they should be able to do with their knowledge become more complex as their grade level increases). To make that determination, teachers provide and interpret both formative and summative assessments, which are often structured, but not always.

Formative assessments are designed to provide a path to improve a student's performance—or at the very least, a benchmark to determine what underlying competencies a student may have (Bloom, Hastings, & Madaus, 1971; Fenwick & Parsons, 2000; Nitko & Brookhart, 2014; Scriven, 1967; Wiggins & McTighe, 2005). For example, college students are often given opportunities to submit drafts of final papers, receive feedback, and revise the submission. That feedback guides students to a better paper or better performance. Formative assessments tend to be ongoing, can be more informal, and are more process oriented. Different types of formative assessments include a simple checklist, an exit ticket, short questions to the class after a lesson, or a teacher watching to see what competencies a student already has.

Summative assessments are designed to make a determination of whether or not a student has mastered or met a competency. Summative assessments are evaluative judgements, often graded, and are product oriented (Bloom, Hastings, & Madaus, 1971; Fenwick & Parsons, 2000; Nitko & Brookhart, 2014; Scriven, 1967; Wiggins & McTighe, 2005). For example, the end-of-week spelling test or the end of the semester final paper will receive a final grade. Testing, whether high-stakes or not, is a form of summative assessment.

Educational interpreters must know the goal of any summative assessment before attempting to interpret it. The following discussion assumes that the

Deaf student has interpreting accommodations for summative assessments documented in their IEP. If they do not, then the educational interpreter should not interpret the content of any summative assessment. If the summative assessment is testing literacy or knowledge of English structures, then that assessment should not be interpreted. If a Deaf student has test items on a literacy assessment interpreted for them, then their responses would not be based on their English literacy skills. However, if the assessment is to determine mastery of a spelling list, how many sides are on a square, who Martin Luther King, Jr. is, or the six simple machines, then test items should be interpreted, provided the Deaf student has appropriate documentation in their IEP.

Interpreting assessments appropriately is easier said than done. As educational interpreters, we need to reflect on what the assessment is trying to measure. Consider, for example, what the Grade 1 assessment in the South Carolina curriculum is addressing:

> SC.1-3.3 Summarize the contributions to democracy that have been made by historic and political figures in the United States, including Benjamin Franklin, Thomas Jefferson, Dorothea Dix, Frederick Douglass, Mary McLeod Bethune, and Franklin D. Roosevelt.
>
> (South Carolina Department of Education, 2011, p. 15)

Do we want students to demonstrate their knowledge of the contributions made by political figures such as Frederick Douglass to democracy? Of course! They may very well know that information but be challenged to demonstrate their knowledge on an assessment because of English fluency. It is important to understand the difference between assessing English language skills and assessing content knowledge. English literacy and bilingual mastery for Deaf students is a significant challenge for a variety of reasons, including language deprivation, a lack of opportunities for direct instruction in ASL in mainstream educational settings, a lack of curriculum designed to meet the literacy needs of Deaf students, and the fact ASL and English do not share the same modality (Arpino, 2022; Briggle, 2005; Caselli, Wyatte, & Henner, 2020; Geers, 2002; Hall, 2017; Haptonstall-Nykaza & Schick, 2007; Marschark & Knoors, 2012; Marschark & Wauters, 2008; Snoddon, Small, & Cripps, 2004; Winston, 1994). If an assessment's intent is to determine whether a student can identify Martin Luther King, Jr. as a civil rights leader and the chronological landmarks of the time period, educational interpreters need to ensure the literacy levels of a Deaf student do not prohibit them from showcasing their mastery of that information. In the case of this example of SC.1–4.3, it would be an appropriate accommodation for a Deaf student to have the test questions and answer options signed to them so that they can showcase their mastery of the content without an English literacy barrier. However, the accommodation of having test questions and answer choices signed must be included in the Deaf student's IEP.

High-Stakes Testing

Students often undergo high-stakes testing as part of their education, which can include standardized tests. These summative assessments hold significant academic consequences for students, particularly since this type of testing can determine whether a student progresses to the next grade, whether a student is on grade level in their academics (system assessment), whether a student passes a course (end-of-course exams or AP tests), and whether the student can graduate. Some high-stakes testing can even make or break college applications, such as the American College Testing (ACT) and Scholastic Assessment Test (SAT).

As an educational interpreter, we have to fully understand what types of accommodations or modifications are allowed during high-stakes testing, and these should be outlined in the Deaf student's IEP. Educational interpreters may prepare for high-stakes testing by requesting a copy of the accommodations page of the IEP so that they know what they are allowed to do. Generally, no exam question can have content altered in any way. However, some exams allow for accommodations such as a distraction-free test location or extended test time.

As we have mentioned, educational interpreters must understand the goal of any assessment, both holistically and for individual test items. However, with any high-stakes testing environment, test security is paramount and very rigid. There may also be specific training the educational interpreter needs to take prior to being allowed access to the test or the testing environment. Educational interpreters may be able to preview the test questions beforehand, but as testing is now primarily done using computers, there is less and less chance that can happen. This results in the educational interpreter having limited access to the test beforehand, which directly affects how well the educational interpreter can determine the goal of each test item.

Some national high-stakes tests will not allow *any* interpreting. For example, an SAT exam will only allow interpreters to be used for oral instructions and not to interpret any test question content. This is partially due to the lack of standardization inherent in interpreting. No two interpreters will sign test questions the exact same way, but test question wording goes through a rigorous process of calibration and validation. If a test item is interpreted differently across Deaf students, it is invalidated and the Deaf students' results can no longer be compared with other test takers'.

SF: I remember interpreting a high-stakes test taken by all grade 4 students in the state to determine the education system assessment. One of the questions involved a music store and the number of compact discs (CDs) in a variety of musical categories such as jazz, classical, and rock. With high-stakes testing, we are absolutely not allowed to change the content in any way—I tend to smirk with the notion of a verbatim (no such thing) interpretation. Suffice to say the Deaf student asked the exam proctor what these types of music categories were. The proctor could not adequately explain types of music. I am confident the Deaf student did not answer the question correctly.

Academic Subjects

Academic subjects are any class or lesson that is taught as part of the school day. These can be typical core classes like English, mathematics, science, and history, or specials/electives which may include physical education, art, and music. For all academic subjects, preparation is key in order to interpret effectively. An educational interpreter must understand the material beforehand. This means that educational interpreters need to have a broad base of general education as well as good study habits. General education classes in college are one option for developing content understanding, but there are an increasing number of options available for learning: YouTube, Khan Academy (Khan Academy, n.d.-a), podcasts, documentaries, books, museums, etc. Find what works for your learning style! In addition to content knowledge, an educational interpreter needs to understand what the lesson objectives are each day. Lesson objectives will come from the state standards and the curriculum, and they are usually also posted somewhere in the classroom.

DC: Algebra was never my strong suit. I failed it in eighth grade and had to retake it in summer school. I still did not understand it well. My first job as an educational interpreter was in a middle school. I paid close attention with my adult brain to the middle school teacher as they taught … and I started to understand it. I would stay after class and ask the teacher questions about the material. I even took the tests with the class since the Deaf student did not have tests signed to them as an accommodation. The Deaf student and I had a little competition going over our test scores, and when they beat me, I would buy them lunch. Find what works for your learning style!

Academic Vocabulary

Many educational interpreters get stressed about knowing the signs for all of the technical and specific words in each academic course. What is more important is to remember that ASL is a compounding language; thus, there is often *not* a one-sign equivalent to many English words. English tends to prefer single words to describe something in detail whereas ASL compounds signs together. For example, BOY + SAME = BROTHER, or STUDENT = LEARN + PERSON. The English language also tends to have discrete words for every nuance of a concept. Think of all the different English words for shades of blue that you know—e.g., azure, cyan, royal, ocean, midnight, sky, navy, turquoise, aqua. Now, think about all the ASL signs for "blue." There is only one sign, BLUE, which is then modified with compounding and nonmanual markers. For instance, different shades of blue might be rendered as follows: BLUE + DARK, BLUE + LIGHT, etc. Shades of blue might also be rendered with a mouth morpheme "shhh" or "ooo" to indicate values of dark or light. While this is a rudimentary example, it again illustrates that ASL is a compounding language, but English is not.

With this in mind, educational interpreters are encouraged not to stress about seeking out extensive, very specific signs for many of the academic subjects' terminology. Instead, focus on understanding what the concept of that English word is, and *sandwich* it with fingerspelling. For example, the word *immigrant* essentially means a person who moves to a new country. To manage that English word, an educational interpreter would want to fingerspell it, provide several signs for that concept, and fingerspell it again. This may look like: I-M-M-I-G-R-A-N-T PERSON MOVE-TO NEW COUNTRY I-M-M-I-G-R-A-N-T (Alawad & Musyoka, 2018; Fitzmaurice, 2024; Haptonstall-Nykaza & Schick, 2007; McKeown, Beck, Omanson, & Pople, 1985; Reutzel & Cooter, 2004; Roos, 2013; Stone, Kartheiser, Hauser, Petitto, & Allen, 2015). Each time the word immigrant comes up, repeat that sandwich process in addition to using formal ASL signs for the concept *immigrant*. These efforts provide the Deaf student the opportunity to understand the meaning of the word and tie it to the printed English word after several exposures. Later, we will discuss in more detail what this looks like. What is key is to recognize that many of the words in academic subjects need to be understood well by the educational interpreter so they can use ASL to convey those concepts while also tying them to the English print.

DC: I worked with a brand-new educational interpreter who was overwhelmed in a middle school science class. The Deaf student was in the class as an opportunity to be with the general education population of students, but they were not on grade level with their peers. The class bell ringer activity was, "How do we know when Easter will be?" The answer to that question is, "Easter is on the first Sunday after the full moon that follows the spring equinox." Even had this educational interpreter known ASL signs for "full moon" and "equinox," the Deaf student would not have known those signs or concepts, so using them without any scaffolding that explained the concepts of full moon and equinox would have been an educational disservice to the student. Even if the interpreter did know the ASL signs for "full moon" and "equinox," they should still use depiction (classifiers) and scaffolding—brief explanations of a concept—in order to be effective.

Why does all this matter? It is important because we hear people state that ASL does not have standardized signs for many technical terms. As a compounding language though, ASL easily conveys the meaning of all those terms, and how to do it is the choice of the signer. Again, we sandwich those compounded signs with fingerspelling. Due to this significant difference in languages, we strongly urge educational interpreters not to stress out about finding the correct sign per se but to get used to treating technical vocabulary as a compounded sandwich, requiring a high degree of fluency and facility with both ASL and the academic subject matter.

Often, we witness less skilled educational interpreters being placed with students enrolled in lower grade levels. The thought behind this practice is that early classwork is less challenging than upper-level classwork. More pragmatically, the thinking stems from the idea that interpreting young children's storybooks or learning simple addition is easier by far than interpreting *Where the Red Fern Grows* or advanced algebra. Such placements result from a misunderstanding of early language acquisition and cognitive development. In fact, younger children need fluent Deaf adult language models, such as Deaf Interpreters or Deaf Language Coaches, in order to build their language foundation (Cawthon, Johnson, Garberoglio, & Schoffstall, 2016; Thibodeau, 2021), as well as skilled educational interpreters who can attempt to minimize the effects of language deprivation while also actively seeking to support the Deaf student in building English literacy (Boys Town National Research Hospital, 2021; National Association of Interpreters in Education, 2019). This is no small factor at all.

Consider, for example, the "simple" task of learning the alphabet. Hearing children have exposure to the sounds of their language and alphabet songs for several years before being asked to learn the actual alphabet—26 individual letters in a specific order that represent, in English, roughly 44 different sounds. For Deaf children from non-signing homes, they do not have previous access to either the sounds of those letters or the letters themselves aside from what they see in the environment on toys, TV, posters, etc. When these Deaf children come to school, they are expected to memorize 26 letters in order—without understanding or having access to the phonemes in English—while mapping those print letters to a visual language system such as ASL fingerspelling, which they may also just be learning. The ABCs are seen as a basic foundational component of literacy, often learned in preschool, and yet this seemingly simple task becomes markedly more difficult for a Deaf student without a complete first language foundation.

From here, we will discuss nuances of some of the major subjects/classes, understanding that the considerations discussed above apply to every single one of these subjects.

English Language Arts (ELA) Classes

Certainly, English Language Arts (ELA) classes are very challenging, both for Deaf students and for educational interpreters. ELA classes in early grades tend to focus on language structure, literacy, and writing. As students move toward higher grade levels in the school system, ELA classes tend to shift focus to types of texts, literature, and poetry.

Spelling, phonics, and phonological awareness in English (rhyming, syllable counting, and sound–letter correspondence) are at the core of elementary ELA classrooms. Hearing children are typically taught reading with items they know; for example, the word "tree." Instruction starts with the sound of the word (for example, /t/, /r/, /i/), then sound–letter correspondence (phonics: T makes a /t/,

R makes a /r/, and EE makes /i/), and then English print (tree). Even if a hearing child cannot spell the word, they have the advantage of sounding it out with their phonics skills. For Deaf students, there is a huge extra step. They must learn the item (tree), the sign TREE (which looks nothing like the fingerspelling), the fingerspelled T-R-E-E, and finally the print "tree."

Deaf students have difficulty developing phonological awareness in English in the same manner as their peers. Hearing aids or cochlear implants do not guarantee full enough access to the sounds of English for Deaf students to develop phonological awareness with the same rate of success as their hearing peers. However, it is important to note that some hearing students also do not learn to read through traditional phonological awareness and phonics. There are approaches to teaching literacy, such as the whole-word approach, that tend to be used as interventions when children fail to read through phonics instruction. As educational interpreters, we know phonics-based strategies often do not work for Deaf children and, rather than expending our interpreting efforts to develop such, we should use literacy strategies that do work. Deaf students can and do learn to read without relying on traditional phonological awareness in English.

There are strategies that educational interpreters can employ in consultation with classroom teachers. These strategies focus on the visual correlates for phonological principles. For example, instead of phonological phenomena such as a focus on rhyming sounds, we can focus on words that have the same print ending. Rather than focus on sound–letter correspondence, we can focus on fingerspelling letter and print letter correspondence (orthographic awareness). Rather than focusing on letter-sound clusters, we can focus on meaningful chunks of words. For Deaf students, word patterns, sight words, and visual memory of words are key skills to develop.

Grammar instruction tends to only appear in the general curriculum until late elementary school, and we must then return to our knowledge that ASL and English are fundamentally different, not just in modality but in their syntax as well. ASL students, and interpreters, struggle with letting go of English grammar when signing. These differences make translating written English concepts into ASL a major hurdle. For example, word order, verb tense, articles, idioms, etc. differ between ASL and English. It is up to educational interpreters and the rest of the IEP Team to figure out how to manage all of this. One strategy that seems to work well for Deaf students is first a conceptual interpretation of the text followed by a more literal interpretation of the text, supplementing all the English grammatical words with fingerspelling but translating the function words. For example, with the sentence: The dog is happy to see you. You would want to sign: DOG-INDEX HAPPY SEE-YOU and then T-H-E DOG I-S HAPPY T-O SEE YOU.

Once students transition into writing assignments, it is difficult for Deaf students to apply the rules of English grammar in their writing. Educational interpreters then need to navigate between both languages, offering visual explanations for English grammar and using fingerspelling (as above) to represent distinctly English grammatical features, and work closely with ELA teachers and IEP Team members to support Deaf students' efforts. Here again, Deaf students have a heavier load than their hearing peers. During writing, hearing students have to translate their thoughts to paper, but Deaf students have to translate their thoughts from one language to another and THEN translate them to paper.

We must inevitably discuss poetry and, by default, rhyming. As you know, poetry often relies on the auditory features of English including rhyme, rhythm, meter, etc. Although ASL does have features of rhyme, rhythm, and meter, the modality difference makes these impossible to translate. Rhyme in ASL is through similarities in handshape, movement, and location. Rhythm is through movement, and meter is through movement and location. Truthfully, auditory rhyme cannot be conveyed well in a visual language, and rhythm and meter can be challenging to represent cross-modally. Certainly, educational interpreters can convey the meaning and emotion behind a poem but cannot convey the basic construct. Educational interpreters will want to work closely with the IEP Team on how to manage interpreting lectures and discussion about poetry. One example is through the use of visual symbols to show meter. By adding stress marks or other symbols to differentiate stressed versus unstressed syllables, Deaf students can rely on what they see to understand the concept of meter. Another example is through the use of orthographic principles to understand rhyme and alliteration. Educational interpreters should be aware of these techniques so that they can collaborate with the IEP Team on the implementation of these principles.

SF: There is a case to be made that the interpretation of any poem to and from any language is simply inefficient and does a disservice to the poem itself. While that is nice in theory, it often doesn't help Deaf students who are held accountable to knowing English poetry. I strongly believe educational interpreters should work with the IEP Team to ensure elements of spoken language (e.g., phonics, poetry) are modified in the IEP to accommodate a visual language. What that means in practice: would time not be better spent having a Deaf student studying ASL poetry?

As students move through different grade levels, vocabulary and sentence structures become more complex—not just in ELA classes but in all classes, particularly in terms of reading comprehension and writing. Educational interpreters will heavily rely on pre-teaching such vocabulary and will use a variety of strategies to make these complex structures more digestible for Deaf students. Again, this work involves the entire IEP Team.

Literature Classes

Literature classes focus on the analysis of literary texts and genres from various places and time periods. Literature analysis requires the use of literary devices such as metaphors, similes, symbolism, irony, and idiomatic expressions, which again do not easily translate into ASL. The best approach for these factors is to use ample classifiers, role-shifts, and storytelling techniques. Such classes also involve promoting a deep analysis of themes, characters, genre, and other such literary structures. As a result, educational interpreters need to unpack a multitude of abstract concepts and convey them in a visual language.

SF: It is often easy for children to learn vocabulary for concrete concepts such as desk, chair, clock, room, dog, or teacher. The more abstract concepts are challenging. The concepts of love, hate, theme, morality, missing someone, justice, or fairness are more difficult. For example, to convey the concept of love, one may use the sign for LOVE which looks like a hug. Does all love involve a hug? Complicated? Indeed.

Like ELA classes, managing interpreting services in Literature classes requires the entire IEP Team to design reasonable expectations, approaches, strategies, and modifications as necessary. For educational interpreters, pre-reading, preteaching, and preparation are critically important.

True of all classes, but of Literature classes in particular, there are class discussions where students are encouraged to share ideas, ask questions, and offer insights. This classroom discourse is an extremely difficult pattern for educational interpreters and Deaf students to follow. Educational interpreters must move around the room to be as near as possible to the hearing student who is speaking; and often students do not speak loudly, clearly, with much coherence, or one at a time. Challenging? Yes. Plus, the Deaf student must also track all the conversations (on a delay). Strategies for educational interpreters in these situations include working with the general education teacher to ensure students understand turn-taking and pacing practices that allow extra time for interpretation, and making efforts to include the Deaf student by directly checking in with them. Educational interpreters can ask for clarity, re-emphasize the importance of turn-taking, and summarize comments as needed.

Another common factor in Literature classes (and really, in most classes) is the use of multimedia materials. These can include audiobooks, movie adaptations, podcasts, YouTube clips, etc. Regardless of whether these materials are captioned or not, as educational interpreters we have an obligation to interpret them. For Deaf students, the three-way attention split of watching the interpreter, captions, and multimedia content is extremely challenging. Over time, Deaf students do become adept at tracking all that input, but it sometimes helps if they are allowed to preview those multimedia materials as part of homework the day before (though this, again, places a greater burden on the Deaf student than on their hearing peers). In addition, educational interpreters can seek out similar content and materials that are presented in ASL. For example, many

Shakespearean plays are available in ASL and/or interpreted. Encourage the general education teacher to use those either for the whole class or, at the very least, as an alternative for the Deaf student.

Math Classes

Math instruction in ASL is highly effective. Deaf children can and do learn mathematics in the same sequence and manner as hearing students. However, most Deaf students lag approximately three years behind hearing students. Again, this is fundamentally attributed to language deprivation and resulting delays. You must have some language foundation to understand mathematics principles. We also note, as there is ample evidence in the research literature, ASL as a language of instruction for mathematics works well. The key to this is the educational interpreters' interpreting abilities alongside their understanding of mathematics.

One of the most frustrating challenges for educational interpreters and Deaf students is the language of math. Much of mathematics teaching relies on talking through problem solving. This sounds like a math teacher saying, "add the ones column and carry over the two to the tens column," or "F of X equals *x* squared minus five," or "for all the values of *x* and if *f* of *a* equals 4, what is one possible value of *a*?" Interpreting this requires a complete visual set-up of the math problem in space, which takes a great deal of time. Instead, we strongly recommend that, rather than interpreting math sentences as such, educational interpreters use a small whiteboard and write out the equation, solving it step by step. Even better, if the teacher is writing out the equation and steps at the front of the room, stand near the board and index the math equations written there as you interpret the discussion. This modeling and repetition are how Deaf students learn mathematical processes. Furthermore, having the problems written out provides immediate context for the actual work of the math problem (i.e., adding, carrying, squaring). This reduces the cognitive load for both the Deaf student and the educational interpreter!

Certainly, specific mathematics vocabulary such as denominator, exponent, or derivative can present a challenge for some educational interpreters. Linking vocabulary with the abstract, symbolic representation of math concepts can be challenging for all students. How does an educational interpreter convey ÷ is the same as / in some contexts, or symbols such as π or √*a*? Deaf students must be able to recognize the terms and symbolic representations on a test. We recommend any educational interpreter study up on their mathematics, both vocabulary and mathematical processes, using appropriate preparation strategies.

Add to all of this, auditory mnemonics in any subject do not work for Deaf students—and serve as just another thing for a Deaf student to memorize. For example, the order of operations mnemonic PEMDAS (some places and generations use BEDMAS): parenthesis (or brackets), exponents, multiplication, division, addition, and subtraction. It helps hearing students to use this mnemonic but, again, it is just another thing for a Deaf student to memorize. Better solutions can be found with your IEP Team, such as writing it out: $()^{2} \times / + -$ written and signed the same way over and over. This creates a visual mnemonic rather than an auditory one.

Educational interpreters also need to keep in mind that general ASL vocabulary does not equate to math vocabulary. For example, the sign DIVIDE makes complete sense in a language-based sentence such as: *The country was divided between red and blue states*. This sign for DIVIDE does not make sense in math, though. Likewise for ADD, EQUALS, SUBTRACT, LESS-THAN, MORE-THAN, etc. We strongly recommend educational interpreters use the graphic symbol to convey math concepts rather than using ASL signs for such. For example, +, =, –, <, >, etc. The effort to match the handshape/sign to the graphic symbol is much more helpful for Deaf students. The Atlanta Area School for the Deaf's Accessible Materials Project (AMPresources, n.d.) has an excellent series of videos with Deaf mathematician Christopher Kurz that provide information on math concepts and signs in context. Khan Academy has also partnered with Rochester Institute of Technology's National Technical Institute for the Deaf on a series of algebra tutorials with Deaf mathematicians (Khan Academy, n.d.-b). Educational interpreters should look to the Deaf community for guidance on how to appropriately convey such information, and resources from Deaf schools and Deaf university programs are one way in which to accomplish this.

A major hurdle for educational interpreters is the pacing and instructional speed of math classes. At lower levels, there are quick, rote memorization features such as choral reciting of even numbers, odd numbers, or multiplication facts. At higher levels, teachers often move quickly through complex material and formulas, which are a challenge to keep pace with while also allowing the Deaf student sufficient time to solve problems in real time. Work with your general education teacher to collaborate in order to mitigate these factors. For example, maybe the entire class can write out the multiplication facts instead of reciting these out loud. Accommodations that the teacher makes for Deaf students will benefit hearing students as well by giving more time for processing as well as additional visual support for auditory materials.

Word problems are a formidable challenge for Deaf students. The relationship between reading comprehension and understanding problem solving in word problems is undeniable. The combination of language comprehension, fraught with idioms, complex sentence structures, and unnecessary details, and the expectation to pair those with mathematical reasoning is also a challenge for many hearing students. For educational interpreters, what is key is to identify and emphasize key words and phrases in ASL in order to help Deaf students recognize those in the printed text. And yes, it is tough to navigate between both English and ASL structures and forms while also ensuring the mathematical bits and pieces are clear. Working with the IEP Team for extra support is extremely important with word problems.

More generally, Mathematics Anxiety (MA), a negative emotion when a person is confronted with math, generally interferes with hearing people's math performance (Ashcraft, 2002; Beilock & Maloney, 2015). Certainly, many Deaf and hearing students experience MA, but it affects Deaf students differently. MA has been found to be higher among Deaf students than hearing students (Ariapooran, 2017; Adigun & Iheme, 2020; Mishra, 2020). For hearing students, negative feelings about math result in high MA, and students often cannot overcome this aversion. For Deaf students though, the opposite effects are evident. Deaf students with more positive feelings toward math had higher MA. Additionally, Deaf students often cannot get any help at home for math homework because of language and communication barriers, and do not have the opportunity to develop math confidence.

Interpreters are often tempted in math class (and in social studies when interpreting geographic information) to interpret from the student's perspective rather than the signer's perspective. When you sign a math sentence (or talk about East/West and right/left directions), you sign from your own perspective and the recipient of your signed message mentally rotates the information to their own perspective. *Mental rotation* is a challenging cognitive task, and it is one that is enhanced in Deaf people, partly because of the use of signer's perspective (Emmorey, Klima, & Hickok, 1998; Janzen, 2006; Talbot & Haude, 1993). Interpreters are tempted to think they are causing confusion for the Deaf student when they use signer's perspective, because it "looks backwards" to the student. However, when interpreters choose to sign math sentences or directions from the student's perspective, they are confounding the Deaf student's language acquisition process of ASL. In ASL, we use signer's perspective for everything. If the interpreter is the language model for the Deaf student and they use structurally inaccurate signing, the student then learns to receive ASL structurally inaccurately and they will be backwards with math sentences and directions. Resist the temptation to sign from the student's perspective. Instead, model how you see the information and show the student repeatedly that you are signing it the way you see it, and that they should sign it the way they see it.

As you have seen, interpreting math classes for Deaf students requires a blend of linguistic precision, visual-spatial interpretation skills, and collaboration with teachers and the IEP Team to manage pacing and content delivery. By addressing these challenges and creating a visually supportive environment, Deaf students can succeed in math classes.

Science Classes

Interpreting science classes for Deaf students presents unique challenges due to the specialized language and the rapid pace of classroom instruction. Similarly to mathematics, the highly specialized terms, formulas, and concepts in science classes are vital for Deaf students to know. Educational interpreters will need to treat each of those terms as key vocabulary and clearly explain these concepts. Pre-teaching key concepts is particularly important in science classes, as lectures often combine demonstrations and multimedia presentations to augment the general instruction. Since humans cannot visually track two different stimuli well, educational interpreters need to allow sufficient time for a Deaf student to look at the demonstration and then watch the interpretation. For educational interpreters, this means holding on to information and often summarizing its key points as opposed to interpreting it all. As with many subjects, there are ample online resources to help with this and, as always, work closely with the IEP Team.

Like math, abstract concepts in science can be difficult to convey in the absence of a direct visual representation. Heavy depiction (classifier) use and good preparation are needed for effective interpretation, along with sandwiching and scaffolding concepts. Educational interpreters must understand science concepts to be able to interpret them effectively. Again, there are multiple sources for studying subject matter in English, and one of our favorite resources for science concepts in ASL is Atomic Hands (Atomic Hands, n.d.).

In terms of labs, educational interpreters, first and foremost, must remain safe. This means, despite how awkward it may feel, if you need to wear lab coats, goggles, masks, etc.—just as students do—please do so. Like many show-and-do approaches in public schools, labs often involve hands-on work where the Deaf student must focus on either the teacher or manipulating equipment while watching the interpreter. Written instructions or visual aids are always helpful in these situations, and interpreting consecutively will likely be required.

In summary, interpreting science classes for Deaf students requires careful planning, collaboration with teachers, and a flexible approach to ensure that complex, abstract, and fast-paced content is communicated effectively.

Related Arts Classes

In all related arts classes, students often multitask—using their hands for art projects, sports, utensils, computers, etc. while also needing to understand instructions. As always, this makes it difficult for Deaf students to simultaneously focus on the interpreter and the task. We strongly suggest working closely with the general education teacher to obtain and use visual aids and help break down tasks into manageable steps with clear pauses for interpreting. Oftentimes, we find interpreting consecutively to be more effective, which also helps Deaf students stay engaged.

Related Arts: Music Classes

Deaf people's relationship with music is unique to the person and can be culturally tumultuous. Music is inherently auditory, relying on sound, pitch, rhythm, melody, and harmony, which are not fully accessible to Deaf students. Music is usually understood as an auditory experience, and music concepts often lack direct equivalents in ASL. For example, conveying notes on a scale through concepts such as steps and half-steps is essentially meaningless for Deaf students, though they can be memorized using sheet music. However, music can be multimodal and thereby also appreciated through the visual and tactile senses.

Research reports that some Deaf people interact with music videos and websites as the music is augmented with strong visual cues. Lyrics help Deaf students understand the artist's intention and interpret the song's meaning—akin to poetry. Rhythm, particularly the bass beat, can be made tactile with the right instruments, volume, and flooring. The key is multimodal engagement, which is extremely challenging in public school music classes.

Placement in a music class as a related art should always be the Deaf student's choice rather than a default from the IEP Team. Music is a rotation in almost every elementary program. If the Deaf student receives pull-out services for SPED or Deaf Ed, music class is a good time to schedule them.

Educational interpreters can convey visual aspects of music, such as rhythm, through clapping or body movements. Some Deaf students may use tactile feedback (like feeling vibrations from instruments) to engage with music. They can use visual tuners to adjust their instruments if they play in a band or orchestra. Educational interpreters can also explain musical concepts in visual terms, such as patterns, tempo, or emotional tone. Again, interpreting choices should be made based on the teacher's goals for the class, and the IEP Team should support accommodations that need to be made for Deaf students participating in music class.

Song signers interpret lyrics into sign language and express musical elements with their bodies and faces to convey the meaning, story, and emotions of a song. However, many Deaf people do not like hearing interpreters conveying music into ASL—particularly as they are often fraught with misinterpretations, inaccurate signing, lack appropriate non-manual markers, and do not convey Deaf cultural norms. Therefore, educational interpreters are strongly encouraged to source ASL versions of songs from Deaf music artists rather than attempting to create their own translations. As a side note: against some popular claims, there is absolutely no evidence that music training benefits speech perception in Deaf students. The bottom line is this: we strongly advocate, unless a Deaf student specifically requests it, the IEP Team should not place Deaf students in music classes.

Related Arts: Art Classes

Art classes often involve hands-on activities where Deaf students are engaged in creating artwork and may have difficulty following interpreted instructions while working with materials. Educational interpreters and art teachers should collaborate to ensure that instructions are delivered visually, perhaps using visual aids, with step-by-step demonstrations and written instructions. Educational interpreters may want to again interpret consecutively and be aware that Deaf students may also need more time to switch between watching the interpreter and focusing on their artwork.

DC: De'VIA is a rich aspect of Deaf culture, and art classes afford an excellent opportunity to incorporate it. I once worked with a student in an art class, and their assignment was to research an artist and write a report on them. I introduced the student to Deaf artists (with the teacher's knowledge, of course). As we were scrolling through images, the student saw "Family Dog" by Susan Dupor and expressed an INSTANT connection to the imagery. The teacher allowed the student to sign their report in ASL as well.

Related Arts: Drama and Theater

Drama classes generally rely on spoken dialogue, vocal intonation, and auditory cues, paired with rehearsals and performances. As all students are focused on acting, it makes for a multitude of interpreting challenges: where to stand, how to have the Deaf student memorize and convey their lines, and how to interpret stage directions. However, it also opens new ways of interpreting theater, such as shadow interpreting all the characters. We recommend educational interpreters work closely with the theater teacher to coordinate visual elements of the performance, such as collaborative performances that incorporate ASL to provide more inclusion. For Deaf students in high school theater, this may provide an unprecedented opportunity to participate in shaping their own access. Educational interpreters and Deaf students may want to look at different Deaf theatre groups for inspiration (Deaf West Theatre, n.d.; National Theatre of the Deaf, n.d.; Deafinitely Theatre, n.d.).

Interpreting related arts classes for Deaf students requires creative problem-solving, collaboration between educational interpreters and teachers, using visual and hands-on strategies, and some ingenuity. With thoughtful planning and some creativity, Deaf students can participate fully in these diverse and engaging subjects.

World Language Classes

There are several complex and nuanced challenges related to interpreting in world language classes. We do not recommend Deaf students take world language classes, rather that they spend time mastering their ASL competencies. However, some Deaf students take world language classes with the goal of developing better fluency in a language's written form and/or to better communicate with their families who speak a language other than English. Working closely with the world language teacher and placing emphasis on the printed form of the language are essential.

If the Deaf student has sufficient auditory input, they may want to attempt to develop some of the world language skills through a combination of lipreading or speech patterns. If an educational interpreter has some knowledge of the world language, that is a bonus and will make the task of interpreting a bit easier. Regardless, extensive preparation is needed for such classes.

Perhaps the best strategy is to use an abundance of fingerspelling (Rochester approach). For the sake of this section, we will use French as the world language to illustrate the point. Educational interpreters should not translate the spoken French into ASL. For example, the French phrase "*Elle joue au tennis*" has an ASL equivalent SHE PLAY TENNIS. This approach does not allow the Deaf student the opportunity to recognize any of the French words. Educational interpreters then must be able to recognize the French words and know how to spell them.

Providing the world language uses a Latin-based alphabet, educational interpreters will also want to treat many of the world language words as key vocabulary using the *sandwich technique* you have already read about. In a world language class, new words are very similar to introducing any new vocabulary and may look like U-N-E P-O-M-M-E APPLEU-N-E P-O-M-M-E. While spelling, the interpreter should mouth the French words *une pomme* while fingerspelling and subsequently signing them.

Many languages have diacritic marks such as å, é, ç, î, ü, and so on. Educational interpreters will need to negotiate with Deaf students how to convey such marks. For example, while fingerspelling *le garçon*, the educational interpreters may want to wiggle the C downward slightly to differentiate it from a conventional, non-accented letter C, or for an é an interpreter could tilt the fingerspelled letter to the right slightly.

Educational interpreters will want to incorporate a lot of mouthing into their interpretation and fingerspelling. If the language teacher moves between the target language and English, you will want to let the Deaf student know.

As you can imagine, it is nearly impossible to fingerspell all these world language words and have them make any sense. Educational interpreters will need to work closely with the IEP Team and classroom teacher to creatively address how to best make a world language class as accessible as possible. There is no quick and easy solution, just a few strategies interpreters can use to model both the source language form and its meaning.

Physical Education (PE) Classes

PE classes are fast-paced and obviously involve physical activity, making it difficult for Deaf students to watch the educational interpreter while simultaneously participating in exercises, sports, or games. Plus, the rapid shifts in team play or rules explanations are very hard to follow. However, Deaf students are quite adept at following what their peers are doing even without understanding the rules. For these reasons, PE classes can be fun, but they can also be isolating. Some Deaf students love PE classes as an opportunity to move around and engage in sports. However, Deaf students have also shared that they generally do not understand what is going on in a PE class and have an overwhelming sense of feeling invisible (Alves & Duarte, 2021; Kurková, Válková, & Scheetz, 2011; Saroja & Priya, 2021).

As such, educational interpreters need to work closely with the PE teacher/coach and teach them, as well as hearing students, some gestures so they may directly communicate with Deaf students (Alfrey & Jeanes, 2023; Berge, 2023; Brimm, 2021; Lawson, 2012; Stinson & Liu, 1999). Such gestures can be beneficial to hearing students as well. This is an example of Deaf Gain—the hand signals in baseball were developed by William "Dummy" Hoy, a Deaf baseball player (Bauman & Murray, 2014; Skutnabb-Kangas, 2014).

Teachers and educational interpreters should also use visual signals (such as flags, hand signs, or lights) to communicate instructions. During activity demonstrations or drills, segmenting classes into smaller groups works toward ensuring the Deaf student understands what is being asked of them. PE teachers should also make sure that the Deaf student has a clear line of sight to the educational interpreter during important instructions, and the educational interpreter should be prepared to move around a lot during PE classes.

Vocational, Career, and Technology Classes

Vocational programs are designed for students to address workplace demands and to use applied learning to develop marketable job skills and work ethics. Most vocational programs center around the following major areas:

- Agriculture, Food, and Natural Resources (agriculture, horticulture, equipment operations, veterinary sciences, animal care)
- Architecture and Construction (carpentry; electricity; heavy equipment operations; heating, ventilation, and air conditioning; plumbing)
- Arts, AV Technology, & Communication (commercial graphics, mechanical design, printing)
- Automotive Technology (collision repair, automotive technology)
- Computer Programming (cybersecurity)
- Health Sciences (dental assisting, medical assisting)
- Hospitality & Tourism (culinary arts, baking)
- Human Services (cosmetology, barbering, early childhood education)
- Manufacturing (machine tool technology, welding, small engine technology)
- Public Safety (firefighting, law enforcement)

Deaf students are often funneled into these types of vocational programs (Cawthon & Leppo, 2013; National Deaf Center on Postsecondary Outcomes, 2019; Palmer, Garberoglio, Chan, Cawthon, & Sales, 2020). Concepts in vocational programs rely heavily on the use of depiction (classifiers). For example, conveying the concept of a caliper measurement of a micron distance on the screw thread of a bolt requires lots of depiction.

Such vocational programs tend to use a teach-and-show style. While a hands-on approach may be ideal for Deaf students, these non-traditional classrooms are challenging for educational interpreters. Part of the educational interpreter's role is to accommodate a visual teaching practice. As with science lab classes, Deaf students cannot look at the interpreter and the visual stimuli at the same time, which means important elements of information are less available to Deaf students. This scenario is particularly true when teachers talk while they are demonstrating something.

Educational interpreters should therefore position themselves as close to the teacher and the object or hands-on element as possible, change placements as needed, change the location of the sign space, interpret consecutively, and use a lot of pointing and indexing. These are all coping strategies usually negotiated between the educational interpreter, the teacher, and the Deaf student.

Educational interpreters cannot address these barriers alone—we need to recruit the teachers' cooperation.

Field Trips and Assemblies

Field trips are, in essence, a blend between academic content and extracurricular activities. Field trips and assemblies are also challenging in terms of calculating position and content. Obviously, if you can visit a field trip location beforehand, it will be helpful—but this is often not practical. It may be helpful to use the internet to gain an understanding of the environment and what some features of the field trip may involve. Look for images, videos, and virtual tours that may be available on the location's website. Ask the teacher for a copy of the field trip itinerary. In addition, ask for any scripts that tour guides will use and request that videos shown on-site have closed captioning. Be prepared to interpret video content, because even captioned materials should be interpreted as well.

School assemblies tend to involve gathering all students, teachers, and sometimes parents and/or guests for a specific purpose. Often these happen in large common areas such as the gymnasium or auditorium. During assemblies, it may be difficult to understand what is being said due to the quality of the sound system. Request scripts and/or agendas in advance. It may also be helpful to understand what the general purpose of the assembly is. For example, for a Spirit week before a homecoming football game, there will invariably be a lot of cheering and yelling to generate school spirit and buzz about the homecoming game. Conversely, a "don't do drugs" assembly will be less frenetic and will have anti-drug information and content (though such assemblies may be skits performed by an outside agency, in which case knowledge of theater interpreting is required).

Musical performances are challenging. If it is an orchestra, there is not much to interpret (and truthfully, not much of value to Deaf students without a large bass section). If there are lyrics, then interpreters should have those well-rehearsed ahead of time in order to interpret them effectively. If the lyrics are in another language, there are two schools of thought. One says find an English translation online and interpret that, and the other says do not translate them at all since hearing students do not have access to the material without knowing the other language. If the music performance is in a gymnasium or another room with flooring that carries sound waves as vibration, request seating for the Deaf student where they can place their feet directly on the floor.

SF: I am more inclined to always translate into English and interpret the material as extra language exposure for a Deaf student, as it is never a bad thing. Plus, hearing students listening to a musical performance in another language at least have something to listen to—a Deaf student does not have a lot to process during such concerts.

Extracurricular Activities

The Individuals with Disabilities Education Act (IDEA) requires accessibility to all components of the educational process, including school-sponsored activities such as extracurricular activities. A large part of the unwritten or hidden curriculum happens outside of the classroom: how to win or lose gracefully, how to take turns on a team, how to work with a team, etc. In a public school, this means all the extracurricular opportunities for Deaf students often require an educational interpreter. These can include school sports, after-school programs, marching band, drama club, journalism club, gay–straight alliance club, chess club, recycle club, and any other club you can think of. Extracurricular activities are not just separate clubs or sports, but include graduation ceremonies, field trips, pep rallies, or even special assemblies.

It is important that educational interpreters consider whether they are suited to the specific extracurricular activity. It is challenging enough to interpret—however, if you do not know anything about expressions such as: false start penalties, a flag right slam and toss, knight to rook five, the difference between stage right and house right, or what a newspaper mast is, you will either need to prepare heavily or have a different interpreter cover that extracurricular activity. Preparation is key to effectively interpreting extracurricular activities. Ensure the entire team collaborates to make the preparation, and resulting interpretation, successful.

Beyond understanding the concepts and lingo of a particular extracurricular activity, the most significant challenge is often where to situate yourself as the interpreter. In the middle of the football field? Hovering over the chess board? The key is to find a place where you can easily be seen by the Deaf student while not interfering with the activity itself or jeopardizing your safety. Interpreting extracurricular activities also often falls outside of the normal work hours and should be compensated outside of that cycle.

SF: I have been on the ice for hockey practice as an interpreter and been slammed backwards into the boards and fallen on my backside often. While hilarious for the team, it also provided a reason for both the Deaf student and their hearing teammates to jointly make fun of me. All in all, a great team bonding experience.

Although access is important, it is also important to allow the Deaf student to relate with hearing students. Sometimes, encouraging direct communication with peers instead of interpreting has a better learning outcome for a Deaf student, particularly during extracurricular activities. For example, encouraging the student to write a note on their cell phone or text back and forth with the school newspaper editor is a lifelong lesson in how to navigate in a hearing world. To be clear, the educational interpreter should still be on hand to interpret as needed.

Summary

In this chapter, we discussed educational discourse, language structure, goals, cohesion, and coherence. We also highlighted the importance of teacher talk or register. This chapter also explained how the curriculum is planned learning experiences for students. In addition to the written curriculum found in educational standards, there is a hidden curriculum, encompassing social norms, values, and behaviors learned in school. Educational interpreters must balance interpreting both types of curricula, though the hidden curriculum often presents more challenges. For Deaf students, there is an expanded core curriculum that addresses additional skills such as communication, advocacy, and technology, which are not part of state standards but are critical for their education. When it comes to testing, educational interpreters must carefully assess whether the test is evaluating content knowledge or English literacy. Deaf students may struggle with English literacy, but that shouldn't prevent them from demonstrating content mastery. High-stakes tests, like standardized exams, may come with limited accommodations, making it crucial for interpreters to navigate the restrictions and ensure students have appropriate support.

We also emphasized the importance of placing highly skilled educational interpreters with younger students to address early academic challenges and mitigate language deprivation. Often, less experienced interpreters are assigned to younger grades due to the assumption that early classwork, like simple storybooks or basic arithmetic, is easier to interpret. However, this approach overlooks the complexities of building foundational language skills and English literacy in Deaf students. Skilled educational interpreters are crucial in early education to help bridge the gap between spoken and visual languages, ensuring Deaf students can develop both language and literacy skills effectively.

Then we delved into interpreting academic subjects, including traditional classes like English, math, science, and history, as well as non-traditional ones like physical education, music, art, drama and theatre, world languages, and vocational courses. Lastly, we discussed managing field trips and assemblies, and interpreting extracurricular activities.

Thought Questions

1 How does the distinction between top-down and bottom-up processing influence an interpretation?
2 How might an interpreter adjust their interpreting strategy when a teacher shifts from lecture to classroom discussion?
3 What are some themes you noted in the discussion about interpreting that were common across different subject matter areas?
4 Reflect on your previous experiences, both in school and in your personal life. What areas of core curriculum do you think will be most difficult for you to interpret? What areas do you think will be easiest? Why?

5 The hidden curriculum in schools often creates situations in which implicit biases can make learning difficult for students. Are there specific instances in which implicit biases or knowledge created challenging situations for you as a student? If so, how might these experiences support your work as an interpreter? If not, how might you recognize any implicit biases that you may have to interpret more effectively?
6 How does the omission of student errors in an interpretation affect a Deaf student's perception of their peers and themselves?
7 Why are music and world language courses so much more difficult for Deaf students to access through an educational interpreter? How might these challenges be overcome?
8 Summarize the challenges educational interpreters face when interpreting standardized tests for Deaf students.
9 Evaluate how interpreting for extracurricular activities and field trips might require different strategies or considerations compared to classroom interpreting.

References

Adigun, O. T., & Iheme, U. M. (2020). Mathematics anxiety among deaf learners: An analysis of predictive factors. *The International Journal of Science, Mathematics and Technology Learning*, 28(1), 1–13.

Alawad, H., & Musyoka, M. (2018). Examining the effectiveness of fingerspelling in improving the vocabulary and literacy skills of deaf students. *Creative Education*, 9 (3), 456–468.

Alfrey, L., & Jeanes, R. (2023). Challenging ableism and the 'disability as problem' discourse: How initial teacher education can support the inclusion of students with a disability in physical education. *Sport, Education and Society*, 28(3), 286–299.

Alsubaie, M. A. (2015). Hidden curriculum as one of current issue of curriculum. *Journal of Education and Practice*, 6(33), 125–128.

Alves, S., & Duarte, E. (2021). The invisible student in physical education classes: Voices from Deaf and hard of hearing students on inclusion. *Journal of Physical Education and Sport*, 21(5), 2512–2519.

AMPresources. (n.d.). Home [YouTube channel]. YouTube. Retrieved May 1, 2025, from https://www.youtube.com/@AMPresources.

Apple, M. W., & King, N. R. (1977). What do schools teach? *Curriculum Inquiry*, 6(4), 341–358.

Ariapooran, S. (2017). Mathematics motivation, anxiety, and performance in female deaf/hard-of-hearing and hearing students. *Communication Disorders Quarterly*, 38(3), 172–178.

Arpino, K. (2022). *Starved for knowledge: The effect of language deprivation and "mainstream" education on deaf accessibility to the United States education system.* Honors Scholar Theses. https://opencommons.uconn.edu/srhonors_theses/861.

Ashcraft, M. H. (2002). Math anxiety: Personal, educational, and cognitive consequences. *Current Directions in Psychological Science*, 11(5), 181–185.

Atomic Hands. (n.d.). Home. https://atomichands.com/.

Bauman, H-D. L., & Murray, J. J. (Eds.) (2014). *Deaf gain: Raising the stakes for human diversity*. Minneapolis: University of Minnesota Press.

Beilock, S. L., & Maloney, E. A. (2015). Math anxiety: A factor in math achievement not to be ignored. *Policy Insights from the Behavioral and Brain Sciences*, 2(1), 4–12.

Berge, S. S. (2023). A shared responsibility for facilitating inclusion in school settings where sign-language interpreting is provided. In L. Gavioli & C. Wadensjö (Eds.), *The Routledge handbook of public service interpreting* (pp. 242–257). London: Routledge.

Bloom, B. S., Hastings, J. T., & Madaus, G. F. (1971). *Handbook on formative and summative evaluation of student learning*. New York: McGraw-Hill.

Bloome, D., Power-Carter, S., Baker, W. D., Castanheira, M. L., Kim, M., & Rowe, L. W. (2022). *Discourse analysis of languaging and literacy events in educational settings: A microethnographic perspective*. New York: Routledge.

Boys Town National Research Hospital. (2021). EIPA written test and content standards. Boys Town, NE: Boys Town National Research Hospital. https://cdn.aglty.io/classroom-interpreting/resources/WrittenTestandContentKnowledgeStandards.pdf.

Briggle, S. J. (2005). Language and literacy development in children who are deaf or hearing impaired. *Kappa Delta Pi Record*, 41(2), 68–71.

Brimm, K. (2021). Interpreters collaborating in K–12 education. In E. A. Winston & S. B. Fitzmaurice (Eds.), *Advances in educational interpreting* (pp. 266–284). Washington, DC: Gallaudet University Press.

Caselli, N., Wyatte, H., & Henner, J. (2020). American Sign Language interpreters in public schools: An illusion of inclusion that perpetuates language deprivation. *Maternal and Child Health Journal*, 24(11), 1323–1329.

Cates, D. (2021). Patterns in EIPA test scores and implications for interpreter education. *Journal of Interpretation*, 29(1), 6. https://digitalcommons.unf.edu/joi/vol29/iss1/6.

Cawthon, S. W., Johnson, P. M., Garberoglio, C. L., & Schoffstall, S. J. (2016). Role models as facilitators of social capital for Deaf individuals: A research synthesis. *American Annals of the Deaf*, 161(2), 115–127.

Cawthon, S., & Leppo, R. (2013). Transition experiences for individuals who are culturally Deaf, deaf, hard of hearing, or deaf-blind. *Journal of Disability Policy Studies*, 24(2), 100–110.

Cazden, C. B. (2001). *Classroom discourse: The language of teaching and learning* (2nd ed.). Cambridge, MA: Harvard University Press.

Deaf West Theatre. (n.d.). Home. https://www.deafwest.org/.

Deafinitely Theatre. (n.d.). About us. https://www.deafinitelytheatre.co.uk/about-us.

Emmorey, K., & Falgier, B. (2004). Conceptual locations and pronominal reference in American Sign Language. *Journal of Psycholinguistic Research*, 33(4), 321–331.

Emmorey, K., & Herzig, M. (2003). Cognitive neuroscience of sign language: Implications for classifier constructions. In K. Emmorey (Ed.), *Perspectives on classifier constructions in signed languages* (pp. 221–246). Mahwah, NJ: Lawrence Erlbaum Associates.

Emmorey, K., Klima, E., & Hickok, G. (1998). Mental rotation within linguistic and non-linguistic domains in users of American Sign Language. *Cognition*, 68(3), 221–246.

Fenwick, T., & Parsons, J. (2000). *The art of evaluation: A handbook for educators and trainers*. Toronto, Ontario: Thompson Educational Publishing, Inc.

Fitzmaurice, S. (2017). Unregulated autonomy: Uncredentialed educational interpreters in rural schools. *American Annals of the Deaf*, 162(3), 253–264.

Fitzmaurice, S. B. (2024). Importance of fingerspelling in education settings. In J. Bentley-Sassaman, R. F. Minor, & S. Fitzmaurice (Eds.), *A survey of American Sign Language/English interpreting settings* (pp. 19–32). OER Commons.

Gee, J. P. (2011). *An introduction to discourse analysis: Theory and method* (3rd ed.). Abingdon: Routledge.

Geers, A (2002). Factors affecting the development of speech, language, and literacy in children with early cochlear implantation. *Language, Speech, and Hearing Services in the School*, 33(3), 172–183.

Hall, W. C. (2017). What you don't know can hurt you: The risk of language deprivation by impairing sign language development in deaf children. *Maternal and Child Health Journal*, 21(5), 961–965.

Halliday, M. A. K., & Hasan, R. (1976). *Cohesion in English*. London: Longman.

Haptonstall-Nykaza, T., & Schick, B. (2007). The transition from fingerspelling to English print: Facilitating English decoding. *Journal of Deaf Studies*, 12(2), 172–183.

Iowa Department of Education. (2019). *The expanded core curriculum for students who are deaf or hard of hearing*. Des Moines: Iowa Department of Education. https://educate.iowa.gov/media/6522/download?inline=.

Jackson, P. W. (1968). *Life in classrooms*. New York: Holt, Rinehart & Winston.

Janzen, T. (2006). Space rotation, perspective shift, and verb morphology in ASL. *Cognitive Linguistics*, 15(2), 149–174.

Joos, M. (1962). *The five clocks*. Bloomington, IN: Indiana University Research Center in Anthropology, Folklore, and Linguistics.

Khan Academy. (n.d.-a). Home. Mountain View, CA: Khan Academy. https://www.khanacademy.org/.

Khan Academy. (n.d.-b). Algebra basics. Mountain View, CA: Khan Academy. https://sgn-us.khanacademy.org/math/algebra-basics.

Kurková, P., Válková, H., & Scheetz, N. (2011). Factors impacting participation of European elite deaf athletes in sport. *Journal of Sports Sciences*, 29(6), 607–618.

Kurz, K. B., & Langer, E. C. (2004). Student perspectives on educational interpreting: Twenty deaf and hard of hearing students offer insights and suggestions. In E. A. Winston (Ed.), *Educational interpreting: How it can succeed* (pp. 9–40). Washington, DC: Gallaudet University Press.

Kurz, K. B., Mullaney, K., & Occhino, C. (2019). Constructed action in American Sign Language: A look at second language learners in a second modality. *Languages*, 4(4), 90.

Langer, E. C., & Schick, B. (2004, October). How accessible is classroom discourse to deaf children using educational interpreters? Paper presented at the Colorado Symposium on Deafness, Language, and Learning, Colorado Springs, CO.

Lawrence, S. (2003). *Interpreter discourse: English to ASL expansion*. Interpreter Preparation Program. Ohlone College, Fremont, CA.

Lawson, H. R. (2012). Inclusion of a deaf student: Collaboration with educators. *VIEWS* (Spring), 26–28.

Lawson, H. R. (2021). Educational interpreters: Facilitating communication or facilitating education? In E. A. Winston & S. B. Fitzmaurice (Eds.), *Advances in educational interpreting* (pp. 245–265). Washington, DC: Gallaudet University Press.

Marschark, M., & Knoors, H. (2012). Educating deaf children: Language, cognition, and learning. *Deafness & Education International*, 14(3), 136–160.

Marschark, M., & Wauters, L. (2008). Language comprehension and learning by deaf students. In M. Marschark & P. C. Hauser (Eds.), *Deaf cognition: Foundations and outcomes* (pp. 309–350). New York: Oxford University Press.

Martin, J. R., & Rose, D. (2008). *Genre relations: Mapping culture*. Sheffield: Equinox Publishing.

McDonough, H., Sticken, E., & Haack, S. (2006). The expanded core curriculum for students who are visually impaired. *Journal of Visual Impairment & Blindness*, 100(10), 587–591.

McKeown, M. G., Beck, I. L., Omanson, R. C., & Pople, M. T. (1985). Some effects of the nature and frequency of vocabulary instruction on the knowledge and use of words. *Reading Research Quarterly*, 20(5), 522–535.

McLeod, S. A. (2023). Hidden curriculum. London: Simply Psychology. https://www.simplypsychology.org/hidden-curriculum.html.

Metzger, M. (1995a). *The paradox of neutrality: A comparison of interpreters' goals with the reality of interactive discourse* (Unpublished doctoral dissertation). Georgetown University, Washington, DC.

Metzger, M. (1995b). Constructed dialogue and constructed action in American Sign Language. In C. Lucas (Ed.), *Sociolinguistics in Deaf communities* (pp. 255–271). Washington, DC: Gallaudet University Press.

Mishra, A. (2020). *Math anxiety in deaf, hard of hearing, and hearing students: Antecedents and outcomes* (Honors thesis, University of Connecticut). Digital Commons @ UConn. https://digitalcommons.lib.uconn.edu/srhonors_theses/746/.

National Association of Interpreters in Education. (2019). Professional guidelines for interpreting in educational settings (1st ed.). Retrieved April 30, 2025, from https://naiedu.org/guidelines/.

National Deaf Center on Postsecondary Outcomes. (2019). Research summarized! Key impact areas. U.S. Department of Education, Office of Special Education Programs. https://nationaldeafcenter.org/wp-content/uploads/2019/04/KeyImpactAreas.pdf.

National Theatre of the Deaf. (n.d.). About us. Washington, DC: National Theatre of the Deaf. https://ntd.org/about-us/.

Nitko, A. J., & Brookhart, S. M. (2014). *Educational assessment of students* (7th ed.). Boston, MA: Pearson.

Notre Dame Learning. (2021). Navigating the hidden curriculum. Notre Dame, IN: University of Notre Dame. https://learning.nd.edu/news/navigating-the-hidden-curriculum/.

Nunan, D. (1991). *Language teaching methodology: A textbook for teachers*. New York: Prentice Hall.

Oliva, G. A., & Risser Lytle, L. (2014). *Turning the tide: Making life better for deaf and hard of hearing schoolchildren*. Washington, DC: Gallaudet University Press.

Palmer, J. L., Garberoglio, C. L., Chan, S. W. H., Cawthon, S. W., & Sales, A. (2020). Deaf people and vocational rehabilitation: Who is being served?Austin: The University of Texas at Austin, National Deaf Center on Postsecondary Outcomes. https://nationaldeafcenter.org/vr-report.

Paltridge, B. (2013). *Discourse analysis: An introduction* (2nd ed.). London: Bloomsbury Academic.

Reutzel, D. R., & Cooter, R. B. (2004). *Teaching children to read: Putting the pieces together*. (4th ed.). Upper Saddle River, NJ: Merrill/Prentice-Hall.

Roos, C. (2013). Young deaf children's fingerspelling in learning to read and write: An ethnographic study in a signing setting. *Deafness & Education International*, 15(3), 149–178.

Roy, C. (2000). *Interpreting as a discourse process*. New York: Oxford University Press.

Saroja, M. M., & Priya, E. M. J. (2021). The invisible student in physical education classes: Voices from Deaf and hard of hearing students on inclusion. *Journal of Physical Education and Sport*, 21(5), 2512–2519.

Scriven, M. (1967). The methodology of evaluation. In R. W. Tyler, R. M. Gagné, & M. Scriven (Eds.), *Perspectives of curriculum evaluation* (pp. 39–83). Richmond, KY: Rand McNally.

Sharpe, T. (2008). How can teacher talk support learning? *Linguistics and Education*, 19 (2), 132–148.

Sinclair, J. M., & Coulthard, R. M. (1975). *Towards an analysis of discourse: The English used by teachers and pupils*. London: Oxford University Press.

Skutnabb-Kangas, T. (2014). Afterword: Implications of deaf gain—linguistic human rights for deaf citizens. In H.-D. L. Bauman & J. J. Murray (Eds.), *Deaf gain: Raising the stakes for human diversity* (pp. 492–502). Minneapolis: University of Minnesota Press.

Smith, M. B. (2013). *More than meets the eye: Revealing the complexities of an interpreted education*. Washington, DC: Gallaudet University Press.

Snoddon, K., Small, A., & Cripps, J. (2004). *A parent guidebook: ASL and early literacy*. Mississauga, Ontario: Ampersand Printing.

South Carolina Department of Education. (2011). South Carolina Social Studies Academic Standards. Columbia, SC: South Carolina Department of Education. Retrieved April 30, 2025, from https://artsandsciences.sc.edu/cege/resources/dailygeog/2011SocialStudiesStandards.pdf.

Stinson, M., & Liu, Y. (1999). Participation of deaf and hard of hearing students in classes with hearing students. *Journal of Deaf Studies and Deaf Education*, 4(3), 191–202.

Stone, A., Kartheiser, G., Hauser, P. C., Petitto, L., & Allen, T. E. (2015). Fingerspelling as a novel gateway into reading fluency in deaf bilinguals. *PLoS ONE*, 10(10), e0139610.

Talbot, K. F., & Haude, R. H. (1993). The relation between sign language skill and spatial visualization ability: Mental rotation of three-dimensional objects. *Perceptual and Motor Skills*, 77(3_suppl), 1387–1391.

Thibodeau, R. (2021). A native-user approach: The value of certified deaf interpreters in K–12 settings. In E. A. Winston & S. B. Fitzmaurice (Eds.), *Advances in educational interpreting* (pp. 31–43). Washington, DC: Gallaudet University Press.

Van Dijk, T. A., & Kintsch, W. (1983). *Strategies of discourse comprehension*. New York: Academic Press.

Wiggins, G., & McTighe, J. (2005). *Understanding by design* (2nd ed.). Alexandria, VA: Association for Supervision and Curriculum Development.

Winston, E. A. (1991). Spatial referencing and cohesion in an American Sign Language text. *Sign Language Studies*, 73, 397–410.

Winston, E. A. (1994). An interpreted education: Inclusion or exclusion? In R. C. Johnson and O. P. Cohen (Eds.), *Implications and complications for deaf students of the full inclusion movement* (pp. 55–62). Gallaudet Research Institute Occasional Paper 94–2. Washington, DC: Gallaudet Research Institute.

Winston, E. A. (2001). Visual inaccessibility: The elephant (blocking the view) in interpreted education. *Odyssey* 2(2), 5–7.

Zaini, S. H., Mokhtar, S. Z., & Nawawi, M. (2010). The effect of graphic organizers on students' learning in school types of graphic organizer. *Malaysian Journal of Educational Technology*, 10, 17–23.

5 Deaf Students

Deaf students in mainstream educational settings face a complex landscape of linguistic, cultural, and systemic challenges that require intentional and informed support. Educational interpreters play a pivotal role in bridging communication gaps, yet their responsibilities extend far beyond simply translating spoken language into sign. They must navigate the intersection of Deaf culture, disability rights, and educational equity while advocating for students who often experience marginalization on multiple fronts—including race, class, gender, and language access. This text explores the evolving role of educational interpreters, emphasizing the importance of cultural competence, collaboration with educational teams, and responsiveness to the diverse needs of Deaf students. From addressing language deprivation to supporting assistive technologies and advocating for systemic change, educational interpreters are uniquely positioned to promote equitable, accessible learning environments that respect and affirm Deaf students' identities.

Understanding Culture and Deaf Cultures

As students of ASL-English interpreting, you have been introduced to Deaf culture and Deaf communities both explicitly—through academic coursework and observations—and implicitly—through interactions, fieldwork, and the lived narratives of Deaf individuals. As you prepare for the unique demands of educational interpreting, it is essential to revisit and deepen your understanding of both general cultural principles and the specific dynamics of Deaf cultures. Cultural competence is not merely academic knowledge; it is a skill set that directly impacts how interpreters facilitate access, build trust, and support identity development for Deaf students.

What Is Culture?

Culture encompasses the shared values, beliefs, customs, behaviors, and communication practices of a group. It guides how people interact, how they view the world, and how they interpret behavior. While all human beings eat, sleep, communicate, and seek shelter, the ways in which these actions are carried out

DOI: 10.4324/9781003423058-5

differ dramatically from one culture to another. These variations are not individual preferences or universal human traits but are socially learned patterns that members of a cultural group accept and pass on.

Culture can be understood in two layers: explicit culture and implicit culture (Hall, 1976). Explicit culture refers to the observable aspects of a group: language, clothing, food, rituals, music, literature, and forms of greeting. These are the things we can see, hear, or touch—often the first signs of difference we recognize. Implicit culture, however, operates below the surface. It includes unspoken rules and deeply held values that govern behavior: attitudes toward authority, notions of personal space, concepts of time, definitions of fairness, ideals of modesty and beauty, work ethic, and even the importance of eye contact. These values are often so ingrained that they feel "natural" to members of the culture, even though they are learned. Our cultural upbringing influences our perspectives and contributes to implicit biases, which affect how we interpret.

As educational interpreters, the challenge is that we often assume our own implicit cultural values are objective truths. This assumption can interfere with our ability to accurately and respectfully interpret across cultures. Developing cultural humility means recognizing that our worldview is shaped by our own cultural experiences—and being willing to examine those assumptions.

Cultural Frameworks and Worldviews

Cultural differences often manifest in predictable ways. For example, there are monochronic cultures and polychronic cultures. Monochronic cultures, such as the United States and many Northern European countries, emphasize punctuality, schedules, and doing one task at a time (Hall, 1983). Interruptions are often seen as rude, and time is treated as linear and limited. The United States' monochronic culture can be seen in the adage that "time is money," and the way in which we talk about time as being "wasted," "spent," "allocated," "saved," etc. In contrast, polychronic cultures (e.g., many Latin American, African, and Middle Eastern cultures) prioritize relationships over schedules. People may handle several things at once, and flexibility with time is not only tolerated but expected. American Deaf culture is polychronic, as evidenced by the humorous use of "Deaf Standard Time (DST)" (Goss, 2003).

Cultures are also individualist or collectivist in nature. In individualist cultures, such as the United States or Australia, autonomy, self-expression, and personal achievement are emphasized. In collectivist cultures, including many Asian, Indigenous, and African cultures, community, group harmony, and shared responsibility take precedence over individual desires (Triandis, 1995). American Deaf culture is a collectivist culture.

There are also past-, present-, and future-oriented cultures. Some cultures look to the past and value tradition and ancestry. Others focus on present experience and daily living, while still others orient themselves toward progress, innovation, and shaping the future (Hofstede, 2001).

Recognizing these cultural dimensions allows educational interpreters to better understand and adapt to the expectations and communication styles of Deaf students from diverse backgrounds.

Language Shapes Thought

Language does more than reflect culture—it shapes how we think. This concept, known as the Sapir–Whorf Hypothesis or linguistic relativity (Lucy, 2001), suggests that the structure and vocabulary of a language influence how its speakers conceptualize the world. For example, in many Inuit languages, there are dozens of words to describe various forms of snow. These distinctions are not simply linguistic quirks; they reflect the central role of snow in Inuit life. There are specific words for falling snow, snow suitable for drinking water, hard-packed snow, slushy seaside snow, and more—each term capturing nuanced meaning shaped by environmental necessity.

Similarly, in American Sign Language (ASL), visual-spatial grammar and facial expressions are not simply "extra"—they are integral to how meaning is conveyed. A single ASL sign can express an entire concept that would require a full English sentence, and facial expressions can indicate tone, grammatical structure, or intensity. The visual-spatial nature of ASL leads to measurable differences between native signers and non-signers in things like visual perceptual span and mental rotation. In this way, ASL is a vivid example of how culture, language, and cognition are deeply intertwined (Klima & Bellugi, 1979).

Enculturation, Acculturation, and Intersectionality

The degree to which a person identifies with or practices the traditions of a culture is referred to as *enculturation*. Some individuals fully internalize the beliefs and behaviors of their culture; others may question, reject, or only partially engage with them—especially if they have grown up in multicultural, bilingual, or displaced contexts. Enculturation happens over time as a person adopts more and more practices and traditions of a culture. People who immigrate to new countries, for example, may engage in *acculturation*, adopting aspects of the dominant culture in order to fit in, survive, or succeed.

In reality, most people do not belong to a single, monolithic culture. Instead, they navigate multiple identities simultaneously such as racial, ethnic, linguistic, gendered, sexual, religious, socio-economic, and more. This concept of *intersectionality* recognizes that people's lived experiences are shaped by the unique ways in which their multiple identities overlap and interact (Crenshaw, 1991; Nash, 2008). For example, a Black Deaf queer student from an immigrant family may face unique barriers and possess unique strengths not shared by Deaf students who are white, hearing-parented, or born in the United States.

As educational interpreters, understanding intersectionality is vital. It prevents us from making assumptions based on a single identity marker, such as Deafness, and encourages us to honor the full humanity and complexity of the students we work with.

Deaf Cultures: Singular or Plural?

Historically, the term "Deaf culture" has been used to describe a unified community of people who share a visual language (such as ASL), cultural norms, and a sense of identity rooted in Deaf experiences. While this framing remains important, it can also obscure the rich diversity within the Deaf world (Lane, Hoffmeister, & Bahan, 1996).

There is not one Deaf community—there are many Deaf communities, shaped by intersections of race, ethnicity, class, gender, geography, education, disability, and immigration status. For example, a Black DeafBlind woman with a college degree may share some experiences with other Black individuals, Deaf individuals, Blind individuals, DeafBlind individuals, women, and college graduates, but she also inhabits a distinct cultural reality born of the intersection of these identities that deserves recognition and respect.

That said, there are some common threads across Deaf communities worldwide. Most culturally Deaf people share:

- A belief in the value and richness of signed language
- A shared history of oppression and resilience
- Distinct norms for attention-getting, turn-taking, and physical space
- Pride in Deaf identity and a sense of belonging to a visual cultural community
- Literary traditions in visual poetry, storytelling, and performance

However, it is important to acknowledge that much of what has historically been taught as "Deaf Culture" in the United States reflects white, middle-class Deaf experiences. Educational interpreters must intentionally study the contributions, histories, and lived experiences of Black Deaf culture, Latinx Deaf culture, Indigenous Deaf traditions, and others to gain a truly inclusive understanding.

Audiological vs. Cultural Models of Deafness

A key distinction in understanding Deaf cultures is the difference between audiological and cultural perspectives on Deafness (Bauman, 2008; Ladd, 2003; Padden & Humphries, 1988). The audiological (or medical) model views Deafness as a deficit—a hearing loss to be fixed, minimized, or hidden through technology, therapy, and assimilation to hearing norms. This perspective often prioritizes speech, lipreading, cochlear implants (CIs), and oral language development, viewing signed language as secondary or even undesirable. The cultural-linguistic model, by contrast, sees Deaf people as members of a linguistic and cultural minority. It values signed languages as natural and complete, and it embraces Deaf identity with pride. In this view, being Deaf is not a disability—it is a difference, like being part of an ethnic group with its own language and customs.

These differing worldviews affect not only how Deaf people are treated by educational institutions, healthcare providers, and policymakers, but also how Deaf individuals see themselves. For interpreters, recognizing and respecting this distinction is critical. Our role is not to impose a model, but to support access, autonomy, and cultural affirmation (Hauser, O'Hearn, McKee, Steider, & Thew, 2010; Leigh, Andrews, & Harris, 2016).

Deaf Cultural Norms in Contrast

Cultural norms within Deaf communities often differ from those of mainstream (typically white, hearing) American culture. For example, while touching another person to get their attention may be taboo in many hearing settings, it is entirely appropriate—and often necessary—within Deaf spaces. Sustained eye gaze is also a key component of visual language. Avoiding eye contact may signal dismissal, disinterest, or disrespect, and breaking eye contact mid-conversation is rude. In visual languages, walking between two signing individuals is acceptable. In fact, pausing or apologizing may be unnecessary or even disruptive. Physical contact, such as hugs, is a normative and valued part of interaction in many Deaf communities (Lane, Hoffmeister, & Bahan, 1996; Leigh, Andrews, & Harris, 2016).

These behaviors are not arbitrary—they arise from the visual nature of signed languages and the communal values that underpin Deaf culture. As interpreters, learning to navigate and respect these norms is essential to building trust and maintaining professional integrity.

Cultural Stewardship in Educational Interpreting

Educational interpreters occupy a unique role—not just as interpreters, but as cultural mediators (Fitzmaurice, 2021). Although hearing educational interpreters cannot claim Deaf identity, we are responsible for ensuring that Deaf students have equitable access to Deaf peers, role models, and cultural resources (Hauser, O'Hearn, McKee, Steider, & Thew, 2010).

Educational interpreters are not members of Deaf culture unless they are themselves Deaf, but they can and should be stewards of Deaf culture in their professional roles—especially when working with Deaf students in mainstream educational settings where Deaf culture is often underrepresented or absent. Stewardship involves respecting, upholding, and supporting access to Deaf culture for students—not owning or representing it. Educational interpreters play a key role in facilitating access to Deaf peers, Deaf role models, and natural ASL use while protecting the cultural space of Deaf students by advocating for linguistic and cultural inclusion. This includes recognizing when Deaf culture is being marginalized or misunderstood and advocating for practices that affirm Deaf students' full linguistic and cultural identities.

In other words, educational interpreters bear some responsibility for ensuring Deaf students maintain access to their culture, language, and identity—a responsibility best described as stewardship. To do this well, we must not only study Deaf culture—but also examine our own cultural frameworks, biases, and assumptions. Cultural competence is not a destination; it is a lifelong journey of humility, reflection, and growth.

Ableism

Certainly, there are an abundance of -isms which identify general ideologies, beliefs, and discrimination. We cannot do them all justice by including them here; however, as educational interpreters, it is critical for you to understand how these forms of discrimination exist within you, your community, your culture, and your language. For the purposes of this book, we believe two forms of social prejudices affect all Deaf students, ableism and audism, in addition to any other forms of discrimination. These directly result in barriers to access, inclusion, and a sense of belonging.

The first one is ableism. Ableism is a set of beliefs that devalue and ultimately discriminate against people with disabilities. The core of this belief is that the disabled person needs to be fixed or helped and it often manifests itself with well-intentioned people.

Many Deaf adults consider themselves as members of a cultural minority and not as disabled. However, according to the Americans with Disabilities Act (ADA) of 1990, audiological deafness is considered a disability that qualifies Deaf people for accommodations and services related to their deafness. In education, this includes interpreter services and other accommodations to make education in mainstream settings accessible to Deaf children. This federal definition of deafness as a disability, and the framing of deafness as a disability within education, give rise to ableist views of Deaf people. As an educational interpreter, you will hear interpreters use phrases such as "help the Deaf student" or even the possessive "my Deaf student." We encourage you to examine the ableist nature of these phrases and to avoid developing a habit of using them.

Audism

The second form of covert discrimination is audism. Under the umbrella of ableism, audism is an attitude based on pathological thinking which results in a negative stigma toward anyone who does not hear or speak. The result is a judgment that places limitations on Deaf individuals. This judgment can show up in subtle ways.

We noted how interpreters will often indicate they are "ASL interpreters" and representing only one language, or "Interpreters for the Deaf" ignoring the non-Deaf participants (Fitzmaurice, 2024). These are subtle audist statements. Interpreters are bilingual and are used by both Deaf and non-Deaf or non-signing parties. Focusing on the Deaf consumer only or on the language used by

Deaf peoples is audist. In other words, interpreters should refer to themselves as ASL-English [educational] interpreters. It is always helpful to remind ourselves that we are present because the hearing person cannot sign. Should it not be, then, that we are interpreters for the hearing?

Certainly, the education system is fraught with notions of audism. For example, the position title "Teacher of the Deaf and Hard of Hearing" has an audiological focus. The education system also continues to emphasize an approach to reading instruction that is based on phonics—an audiological route to literacy (Hoover & Gough, 1990). Requiring students to take music as a related arts class or only offering spoken languages as world language credit in different states are audist policies. There are audist perspectives also embedded in assessment settings. For instance, when a test question is phrased as "Describe your favorite music artist," the test question is written with the assumption that the test taker has an ability to hear. All these systemic factors coalesce around audism, or giving preference to the ability to hear.

DC: One of the most insidious types of audism I have seen in education comes from decisions IEP (Individualized Education Program) Teams make about Deaf child language use. I have worked with multiple parents who have had to fight for their Deaf child's right to direct instruction in ASL, educational interpreter services, ASL language assessments, etc. IEP Teams push back on these requests, especially if the child uses cochlear implants and has any semblance of spoken English. However, I have never once seen a team push back against speech language pathologist (SLP) services, school-provided audiological equipment, or any other accommodation designed to prioritize spoken language.

Racism

The social prejudice that affects students of color, and overwhelmingly Black Deaf students, is racism. Racism is the discrimination against another person on the basis of race or ethnicity. Hand in hand with racism are colorism, shadeism, and anti-blackness, which specifically refer to discrimination on the basis of skin tone. Research shows a few concerning trends, particularly for Black Deaf students. One incredibly disturbing trend is the significantly higher rates of suspension and expulsion for Black Deaf students as compared to white Deaf students (United States Government Accountability Office, 2018). These findings highlight systemic inequities and suggest that implicit bias and structural racism contribute to these disproportionalities. Education systems must examine their discipline policies and practices to address racial injustice and promote equitable outcomes for all students.

Another concern the field of ASL-English interpreting needs to address is that a disproportionate number of interpreters are white, thereby reflecting a lack of representation of people of color working as interpreters (Registry of Interpreters for the Deaf, 2018; Stewart, 2020). Consider how we discussed above the educational interpreter's stewardship of Deaf cultures and languages and how it is the interpreter's obligation to ensure Deaf students have Deaf role models (Cawthon, Johnson, Garberoglio, & Schoffstall, 2016).

Famous Deaf faces are far more often white than they are Black. The Deaf history told in Deaf culture classes is white Deaf history. Therefore, educational interpreters again, as stewards supporting Deaf students with maintaining access to their culture, language, and identity, need to be intentional about exposing themselves and Deaf students of color to Deaf members of other systematically minoritized groups. We suggest you start by referring to organizations and resources such as Deaf Women of Color, the National Black Deaf Association (NBDA), and the HeART of Deaf Culture.

Furthermore, the prevalence of white interpreters means that Black Deaf students are not exposed to Black ASL, a known dialect of ASL used within the Black Deaf community (McCaskill, Lucas, Bayley, & Hill, 2011). It also means that Indigenous Deaf students do not have access to their respective language dialects such as Plains Indian Sign Language among others (Davis, 2010; Farnell, 1995; Kendon, 1988; Zeshan & de Vos, 2012). It also means Deaf students from underrepresented backgrounds do not have culturally appropriate interpreters to represent them in their educational environments. Again, as stewards, educational interpreters have some responsibility to ensure diverse Deaf students have access to their respective culture, language, and identity. Therefore, educational interpreters need to be aware of these considerations, recognize the impact they have on the social-emotional well-being of Black, Indigenous, students of color and seek out resources to support diverse Deaf students (The Diversity Academy, 2025).

Narratives of Experience

An interpreted education is not optimal for Deaf students (Antia, Jones, Reed, & Kreimeyer, 2009; LaBue, 1998; Marschark, Sapere, Convertino, & Pelz, 2008; Schick, Williams, & Kupermintz, 2006; Schick, 2004; Winston, 1985; 1990; 1994). Direct instruction by fluent teachers is by far the better and more effective instructional approach for Deaf students (Cates & Delkamiller, 2021; Kurz, Schick, & Hauser, 2015). However, parents ultimately often decide that placing their Deaf child in a mainstream school with an educational interpreter is the better decision for their family. We are not going to debate whether parents have all the information to make such decisions; rather, we are going to share Deaf students' thoughts and experiences about an interpreted education and the educational interpreters with whom they work.

Students recognize the change in roles of educational interpreters from elementary to high school, and they report in early grades that educational interpreters tutor more and generally offer more help. By high school age, students report that educational interpreters adhere to a more traditional interpreting role metaphor (Kurz & Langer, 2004; Russell, 2008). Deaf college adults share three "roles" educational interpreters tend to enact: namely, the roles of friend, teacher, and mentor/parent (McCray, 2013). This is challenging in that educational interpreters should support Deaf students with making connections with hearing students and adults and not be the student's primary, and sometimes sole, connection (Prinzi, 2023; Wolters, Knoors, Cillessen, & Verhoeven, 2012).

Some Deaf students alarmingly report that the least skilled educational interpreters were often placed in elementary school grades (Russell & McLeod, 2009). This is a significant concern, as younger children need very highly qualified, ASL-fluent educational interpreters to minimize the effects of language deprivation (see chapters four and six). Indeed, in the interpreting field as a whole, educational interpreters need access to more training and skill development to be qualified to interpret for both very young children and higher-level academic content.

Recommendations from Deaf students for educational interpreters based on their experiences are abundant. For example, Deaf students want educational interpreters to allow the Deaf student to make their own decisions (Kurz & Langer, 2004; Russell, 2008; Oliva & Risser Lytle, 2014). While educational interpreters should advocate on behalf of students, Deaf students also ask educational interpreters to not coddle (mother) or discipline them and allow students their own space (Hands & Voices, n.d.; National Deaf Center on Postsecondary Outcomes, n.d.-a). This is historically a challenge for some educational interpreters as individuals who are apt to work with Deaf children have "tender hearts" or a "savior complex" and are often tempted to overindulge students. This is further compounded when an educational interpreter works with the same student from preschool through senior year of high school.

Deaf students also appreciate when educational interpreters advocate for them in times where they cannot advocate for themselves. It is also incumbent on the educational interpreter to teach self-advocacy skills and allow Deaf students the opportunities to practice those self-advocacy skills (Fitzmaurice, 2021). Deaf college students overwhelmingly wanted their educational interpreters to demonstrate positive attitudes toward Deaf people and to be knowledgeable about Deaf cultures (McCray, 2013). While this text does not get into the specifics of such, most interpreter programs have such coursework and competencies in their respective curricula. It is important to note that, although a Deaf student may be developing their own identity as a Deaf person, if an educational interpreter is not demonstrating a positive outlook on Deaf people (think high standards), such attitudes can and will "rub off" on the Deaf student.

DC: I worked with an interpreter who worked with a Deaf student in middle school. This student used spoken English expressively their entire elementary education. Then, in eighth grade, they decided to stop wearing amplification devices and to use ASL expressively. Not surprisingly, this coincided with increased contact with Deaf peers. This interpreter refused to interpret from ASL to English for this student because "they can speak for themselves." Don't be that interpreter.

Researchers have also found that Deaf students lament educational interpreters behaving like a "pseudo-parent" by telling students to pay attention and correcting student behavior (Kurz & Langer, 2004; Oliva & Risser Lytle, 2014). There is a fine line between acting as an educator and providing direct instruction (Fitzmaurice, 2021) and becoming parent-like. Again, to avoid these concerns, educational interpreters must work to avoid overstepping the fine line between advocating on behalf of Deaf students and over-nurturing Deaf students.

There is no doubt humans need connection, and Deaf students and educational interpreters will connect in a friendly way (Prinzi, 2023). However, educational interpreters are not truly a Deaf student's friend (Fitzmaurice, 2021) and should be constantly working to foster connections between Deaf and hearing students. Too often, Deaf students become passive recipients rather than full, active participants in their own learning process because of limited social connections besides the educational interpreter, and because well-meaning adults step in and do too much for them.

These reflections and suggestions are critically important, as educational interpreters play a significant role in each student's success.

Deaf Students' Readiness to Learn via Interpreting

Social, psychological, linguistic, and academic development is interwoven. Partly due to this, there is very little research on how learning through an educational interpreter may influence the cognition of Deaf students (Knoors & Marschark, 2014; Schick, 2008). There is also great power in incidental learning (Hopper, 2025; Lederberg, Schick, & Spencer, 2013; Marschark & Knoors, 2015), socialization, and the unwritten curriculum in a school environment (Mitchell & Karchmer, 2012; Musselman, Mootilal, & MacKay, 1996). These are just a few of the challenges with educational interpreting and learning through an interpreted education.

Truthfully, there is little evidence to guide educational teams in terms of whether or not a student is ready for and capable of learning through an educational interpreter. In fact, using an educational interpreter without addressing underlying language deprivation prolongs and perpetuates the deprivation. Language deprivation and its impact are discussed in more detail in chapter six.

Deaf students without a foundational language base cannot fully benefit from the services of an educational interpreter, as language acquisition does not occur through interpretation alone. Learning any language requires rich, interactive, and direct communication—something that the interpreted classroom environment cannot provide. While interpreting provides access to content, it is not a substitute for natural language development. Moreover, educational interpreters cannot function as effective language models during interpretation, as the input is one-directional, lacks interaction, and is often fragmented (Peterson & Monikowski, 2010; Schick, 2004; 2008).

There are a multitude of language assessments that can be conducted by professionals trained in language assessment. Such assessments include the

Kendall ASL Skills Checklist for Kindergarten (ages 5–6), *Standardized Visual Communication Sign Language Checklist*, and the *Language First American Sign Language Receptive Skills Test* (Anderson, 2022; Enns, Zimmer, Boudreault, Rabu, & Broszeit, 2013; Hall-Katter, Leffler, & Perez, 2020; Simms, Baker, & Clark, 2013). These language assessments generally apply to Deaf children from infancy to third grade and provide an accurate picture of their current language levels.

If a Deaf student has sufficient language abilities, they may benefit from using an educational interpreter. They must be able to demonstrate some evidence that they can identify the interpreter as not being the teacher. They must be able to understand that interpreters sign for non-signers. Students who benefit from an interpreter also begin to attend to an interpreter during obvious class discussions, and will maintain eye contact appropriately during interpreted situations. Generally, with enough language and a formed Theory of Mind (see chapter six), these signs of readiness occur around the third grade. Before the third grade, a child generally does not have the cognitive ability nor the language skills to understand the difference between an interpreter and the person for whom the interpreter is interpreting.

Additional clues indicating that a student is ready to use an educational interpreter include:

- Begins to ask questions about signs that are new
- Clarifies signs with interpreter
- Starts to direct content questions to the teacher
- Uses non-manual markers to convey comprehension
- Begins to use an interpreter to talk to classmates on a regular basis, etc.

These are all clear indicators that a Deaf student is ready to use, and can benefit from, an educational interpreter. Naturally, these skills grow stronger as a Deaf student gains experience of working with an educational interpreter. For Deaf students with language deprivation, you will want to advocate using a Deaf interpreter or a language coach rather than an educational interpreter, at least until such time as the Deaf student exhibits readiness for educational interpreter services.

Language Coaches

There is, without a doubt, a lack of Deaf role models for Deaf students in public schools (Cawthon, Johnson, Garberoglio, & Schoffstall, 2016; Johnson, Liddell, & Erting, 1994; Mowry, 1994). This factor alone tends to further isolate Deaf students as they have no aspirational muse and may very well wonder, “Can Deaf people be successful?” and, “Am I the only Deaf person?” Anecdotally, some Deaf children grow up believing they will either die in childhood or become hearing in adulthood because they have not met a Deaf adult.

For the purposes of this chapter, we will use "language coach" to describe a person who provides direct language support for Deaf students, guiding them to acquire ASL fluency. Language coaches engage students in one-on-one and group interactions, modeling language, and supporting the development of cognitive and academic language skills in a Deaf-friendly environment.

Many school systems use different terms for staff such as "language facilitator." Language coaches address the need for Deaf role models and provide a strong, necessary direct intervention to support language acquisition for language-deprived Deaf children.

Language coaches do this by providing a structured, explicit approach to acquiring language through direct developmental language acquisition strategies. Language coaches are fluent in ASL (typically Deaf individuals with ASL as their first language) and are used to address the urgent need for Deaf children to acquire a first language as soon as possible. Generally, an educational interpreter with an Educational Interpreter Performance Assessment (EIPA) 4.0+ score may have the language abilities to provide language coaching services; however, the qualifications and work of an educational interpreter differ greatly from those of a language coach, and a hearing educational interpreter cannot provide the same cultural aspects as a Deaf language coach. Language coaches generally have advanced training in language development, understand the progressive levels of language acquisition and cognitive development, and work to immerse the Deaf child in a natural language environment (Cerney, 2007).

Language coaches can support Deaf students in making significant gains in both their expressive and receptive language (Lederberg, Schick, & Spencer, 2013; Watkins, Pittman, & Walden, 1998; Dostal & Wolbers, 2014). Only after Deaf children achieve sufficient fluency in a signed language do they have the metalinguistic ability to use language in various situations and benefit from an educational interpreter to access their school experience. If a Deaf child does not have a strong language foundation, a language coach should be used for the first few years of school until there is enough language fluency for the Deaf student to transition into using an educational interpreter.

Deaf Interpreters

Deaf interpreters in public schools are effective in both self-contained classrooms and mainstream classrooms alongside a hearing interpreter. Despite a long history of research (Holcomb & Smith, 2018; Thibodeau, 2021), Deaf interpreters have not been widely adopted. Deaf interpreters provide several benefits, not the least of which is that the Deaf interpreter is a good role model for Deaf students (Kurz, 2023; Holcomb & Smith, 2018).

A Deaf interpreter also brings a distinct set of formative linguistic, cultural, and lived experiences as a Deaf person that enables nuanced comprehension and promotes self-determination and autonomy for Deaf students. Their lived experiences in educational settings inform their interpreting schemas. This may include growing up with educational interpreters, expanding and clarifying content for Deaf peers in school, using interpreters with various communication styles, learning strategies they have developed (e.g., dual task management), and a lifetime of navigating the world as a Deaf person. A Deaf interpreter can easily transmit these experiences to Deaf students.

Typically, in mainstream classrooms, Deaf interpreters work at the front of the room (with the teacher) while the hearing educational interpreter is closer to the back of the room interpreting the information (called feeding) to the Deaf interpreter. Another arrangement may be to have the educational interpreter at the front of the room (with the teacher) while the Deaf interpreter sits next to the Deaf student. This allows the Deaf interpreter the ability to provide clarification or summarize what the educational interpreter interprets. In this set-up, the Deaf interpreter can also monitor the hearing interpreter and provide feedback or suggestions (Thibodeau, 2021).

In self-contained classrooms, the Deaf interpreter will often work with the teacher of the Deaf, assisting with language presentation, schema building, connecting cultural contexts, and expansions on concepts (Kurz, 2023; Thibodeau, 2021).

There are several video examples of working with Deaf interpreters (ASLized!, 2014; Center for Atypical Language, 2022a; 2022b). In general, Deaf interpreters are particularly necessary for Deaf students who have language deprivation or those who use a foreign signed language.

Interpreting with Students that Use Hearing Aids

For this text, we have been using the term "Deaf student" for any student who uses signed language to access the education system. We remind you as you read these next sections that we have a cultural view of Deaf people. Deaf people do not need to be fixed or made to use the same language modality as hearing people. Audiological interventions are an incredibly personal decision, and Deaf children should be afforded autonomy in decisions about their use of hearing-assistive technology.

Audiologically, most students are not profoundly deaf and have varying levels of hearing. Educational interpreters should consult with the education team and/or audiologist to see a particular student's audiogram (a graphic representation of a student's hearing levels) and hearing level pattern. This estimates how much a student can depend on hearing to access spoken language and classroom content.

Students may use hearing aids to augment their hearing. While hearing aids amplify sounds, they cannot correct hearing levels and students will still miss a great deal of information—particularly in noisy environments. Often, educational interpreters are by default responsible for ensuring a young student's hearing aids are working correctly. This can include checking and changing batteries, unclogging ear molds, and other such minor actions. All educational interpreters should consult with appropriate members of the team to learn how to do this.

DC: Educational interpreters may be asked to hold onto hearing aids during sports if students sweat excessively, or if they will be swimming. Encourage the student to have their hearing aid or cochlear case on hand during sports so that there is a safe way to store them, and work with the student and teacher to identify a secure place where the technology can be stored. I will never forget being handed a pair of hearing aids at a waterpark (field trip) and seeing all of the earwax on them. Gross.

Educational interpreters should note that students may have an audiogram profile that shifts. For example, educational interpreters may need to adjust their interpreting based on whether the environment is quieter or noisier. If a student has a cold or ear infection, they may temporarily lose some residual hearing. Students may also have progressive loss or fluctuating hearing levels, in which case there will be ongoing changes to what the student can and will access through audition.

Interpreting for Students that Use CIs

CIs are complex electronic devices surgically implanted under the skin behind the ear, designed to provide a facsimile of sound to the human brain. These devices use electrodes placed in the inner ear (the cochlea) to stimulate the auditory nerve of people with significant, permanent deafness. These signals are not equivalent to biological hearing and the greatest challenge is the Deaf child's need for extensive training to develop skills in listening and decoding what they may hear as meaningful *language*.

The abilities of an implanted child to hear with understanding and to speak with intelligibility vary from child to child. Some CIs are more successful than others at electronically processing sound. Because of this, Deaf students with CIs may have enough *auditory discrimination* to begin to understand *some spoken language*. Unfortunately, it is difficult to predict how well a child's brain can interpret the new auditory signals it is receiving with the implant. Not all causes of deafness can be addressed by CIs. Again, a CI does not restore normal hearing; rather, it can provide a useful representation of sounds in the environment and *may* help a Deaf student understand some speech.

Research indicates over half of elementary-aged Deaf children with CIs had spoken language skills below the 16th percentile (that is, significantly below average) (Wie, von Koss Torkildsen, Schauber, Busch, & Litovsky, 2020; Gagnon, Eskridge, Brown, & Park, 2021; Geers, Tobey, Moog, & Brenner, 2008). This means that even with a CI, Deaf children are still at risk for language deprivation due to the lack of exposure to a fully accessible language. In some ways, the risk is even greater because of the assumption parents and educators make that the implant "fixes" the child's hearing and so they resist the introduction of a signed language longer than they otherwise might (Mukari, Ling, & Ghani, 2007).

Likewise, when interpreting with students with hearing aids, educational interpreters will want to learn about the external parts of the implant. For young children, educational interpreters may need to ensure it is attached and that the batteries are charged. Some external parts may need to be removed for some activities, like physical education. If the implant is not connected or has been removed, the child will have no hearing at all—a byproduct of implant surgery (though modern developments allow for the preservation of some residual hearing with some devices).

It is important for educational interpreters to work with the educational team to understand the student's auditory access, use of spoken English, use of ASL, and the educational goals surrounding the use of spoken and signed language. For example, some students may need more interpreting in noisy or academic environments but need less interpreting in social situations where they can practice their listening and speaking skills. Again, remember to keep language and modality distinct in these discussions, and respect the Deaf student's autonomy in their decision making.

Like for students who use hearing aids, a student with a CI may be receiving some of the teacher's spoken message while also watching the interpreted message. Educational interpreters may then need to ensure they interpret in subject-verb-object word order. However, just because a student may not always attend to the interpreter (using their hearing), educational interpreters should continue to interpret so the child can immediately refer to the interpreter for timely clarification.

Deaf-And

The term Deaf-And (in some communities "DeafPlus" or "DeafDisabled") refers to Deaf people with co-occurring disabilities including learning differences, intellectual differences, autism spectrum differences, and Deaf-Blindness. As a result, Deaf-And students use a multitude of different communication systems and tend to have significantly different needs than students who are not Deaf-And.

For example, Deaf-And students with cerebral palsy, Down syndrome, and/or autism spectrum differences might have different language processing or production capacities. Given the role conflict of working as an educational interpreter contrasted with the multitude of other services such students need, IEP Teams should seriously consider whether interpreting services are best for Deaf-And students or if other configurations would be more appropriate (Singer, Cacciato, Kamenakis, & Shapiro, 2020).

Depending on the co-occurring disability, Deaf-And students may experience inattention, impulsivity, and other traits which make interpreting more challenging for both the student and the interpreter. Literacy development will likely become even more challenging too, as Deaf-And students will have different learning needs (Paul, 2020).

For any Deaf-And student, the educational interpreter will have to work closely with the IEP Team to determine if educational interpreting is the best support for that specific student, and/or determine what modifications and additional supports need to be implemented. Most teachers of the Deaf have no specific training for working with Deaf-And students (Guardino, 2015). If an educational interpreter is placed with a Deaf-And student, they will need significant professional development to learn effective practices for meeting the specific needs of that Deaf-And student.

DeafBlind

For students with DeafBlindness, often a result of Usher's syndrome, educational interpreters will need to use several adapted interpreting techniques. Educational interpreters are often the first to notice a Deaf student exhibiting early symptoms of DeafBlindness. DeafBlind students may be completely blind, legally blind, have a restricted visual field, or have functional use of some vision. They may be profoundly deaf or audiologically hard of hearing.

In addition to interpreting language, educational interpreters will also need to provide environmental information for DeafBlind students. For example, describing the room and how it is set up, who is in the room and where they are in relation to the DeafBlind student, always including the speaker's name before interpreting for them, providing the "mood" of the room (e.g., everyone is smiling, or tense), interpreting non-verbal information (e.g., the student beside you is on their phone, the teacher keeps looking at the clock, etc.)—this is all relevant environmental information. Educational interpreters may also be asked to serve as a sighted guide when working with DeafBlind students. This generally means guiding the DeafBlind student to the cafeteria, to the restroom, to the bus line, and so forth.

DeafBlind students may also need adapted communication methods for interpreting purposes, and educational interpreters will want to be extra-sensitive in considering seating, lighting, background, and clothing when interpreting for DeafBlind students. This may seem an odd thing to consider, but educational interpreters will also want to practice good oral hygiene and avoid using strong perfumes or colognes because they will work in close proximity with the DeafBlind student. In terms of interpreting, DeafBlind students may use a variety of adaptations. For example, close vision interpreting is where the educational interpreter sits close to the DeafBlind student and significantly reduces their signing space. Tracking means the DeafBlind student places their hands on the educational interpreter's forearms to help keep signs within their individual vision field.

For DeafBlind students with no functional residual vision, tactile signed language may be needed, which means the DeafBlind student will place their hands on top of the educational interpreter's hands to receive the incoming message. There are a variety of forms of tactile signed language including ProTactile ASL (DeafBlind Interpreting National Training and Resource Center, n.d.; Nuccio

& Clark, 2020). ProTactile ASL requires specific training that may not be available in every state, but it is the language of the DeafBlind community in the United States and it is the most completely accessible tactile language. As with all Deaf-And students, educational interpreters will want to seek additional training on how to work with this population of students.

Immigrants and Refugees

It is challenging for educational interpreters to work with emergent signers in the face of significant language delays (Miner, 2021). As we have touched on repeatedly in this text, interpreting for K-12 students without a language foundation is not feasible because the ability to use interpreting services requires students to have a foundational, functional language. However, most Deaf students have some effects of language deprivation and they are compounded when Deaf students are newly immigrated to the United States or are refugees (Fischbeck, 2021).

Interpreting for such students is particularly challenging given their unique linguistic and lived experiences. There are a number of strategies educational interpreters use to support Deaf refugee and immigrant students (Fischbeck, 2021). In brief, educational interpreters modify their expressive language use by increasing natural gestures and using a significant number of visual aids. These strategies mirror those that educational interpreters use for students with language deprivation. In the case of immigrant or refugee children who use a different signed language, educational interpreters will need to work with qualified Deaf interpreters.

Immigrant and refugee students (and families) may also need support acclimating to the school environment and to the United States as a whole, particularly regarding the IEP process. Educational interpreters should be aware that parents may not know how to navigate the system, may have insufficient access to interpreters, may fear retribution from the system, and may have different attitudes about deafness.

All the Other Tech

Technology is increasingly dominant in mainstream American society, and we as a society are increasingly dependent upon it. Similarly, Deaf people use a multitude of tech to thrive/survive, smartphones notwithstanding. It is important that educational interpreters understand each of the devices Deaf students may need and/or use and how these devices may influence the Deaf student's performance. Additionally, some Deaf students may not have some of this technology in school or at home and it is incumbent on the educational interpreters to advocate for such.

Hearing Aids

Hearing aids are small electronic devices that help hard-of-hearing students hear some sounds more clearly. Generally, there are three main parts: a microphone, an amplifier, and a speaker. Some hearing aids can also reduce background noises as opposed to amplifying all sounds. Modern hearing aids can be customized to a person's specific audiogram and can also include features like Bluetooth connectivity, rechargeable batteries, and even smartphone apps for control and adjustment.

Educational interpreters should know the different types of hearing aids and how they are worn. Some hearing aids are called in-the-ear (ITE) hearing aids, which have a molded case that fits the entire hearing aid in the ear. Behind-the-ear (BTE) hearing aids are common and easier to see. They offer the highest amount of amplification and are frequently used with hard-of-hearing students. BTE hearing aids sit behind the ear and the shell houses the electronics, battery, and controls. A thin tube conducts the sound from the BTE shell to an earpiece that fits in the ear. Bone-anchored hearing aids (BAHAs) are surgically implanted. They may partially restore some types of hearing by using vibrations through the skull bone to send sounds to the ear. These are similar in concept to bone conduction headphones and are often an alternative to CIs for students whose cochlea is improperly formed.

SF: As someone who uses two BTE hearing aids, it is important for educational interpreters to remember that a hearing aid does not completely fix reduced hearing levels like eyeglasses do for vision. Hearing aids only amplify sound but will not make the sound any clearer—just louder. The microphone picks up everything—a breeze can sound like a tornado in a hearing aid microphone. Not all hearing aids suppress all the background noise—for example, dishes and silverware clattering or an air conditioning unit get amplified. Again, this makes using hearing aids a less-than-perfect solution. Lastly, just like hard-of-hearing students, if I have a bout of allergies or a head cold, my hearing levels drop too. My hearing ability is not static and can sometimes go down.

Educational interpreters working with young children may need to help students charge their hearing aids at the end of the school day, help keep them clean, and sometimes be somewhat of an "Are you wearing your hearing aids?" monitor if it is mandated in the IEP. Again, consult with the educational team on how to do this, and always respect the Deaf student's bodily autonomy if they do not want to wear their devices.

CIs

Many Deaf students use CIs, which are electronic devices that are surgically implanted and designed to send electronic signals directly to the auditory nerve. The external component looks similar to a BTE hearing aid and houses the microphone, speech processor, and transmitter. The internal component is implanted under the skin and includes a receiver and electrodes that stimulate the auditory nerve. CIs help students to perceive sound, but outcomes vary significantly in terms of how effective that sound perception may be in comprehending speech. We strongly recommend educational interpreters do a web search on how a CI works and what it sounds like to hear through a CI.

Historically, there is much animosity between the Deaf community and medical practitioners about trying to "fix Deaf people." This argument has waned significantly over the years and the vast majority of Deaf students are implanted. Like hearing aids, sometimes younger children may need some assistance from an educational interpreter on battery changes and keeping their CI clean.

DC: One thing I will never do is force a child to wear a CI or a hearing aid. It violates their autonomy, which is a violation of the first tenet of the Educational Interpreter Code of Ethics. If you are working with a student who is constantly refusing to wear their devices (not forgetting—refusing), but their IEP states they must wear them, that is a good time for an IEP Team discussion about changing that language either to allow for breaks from wearing devices or changing to "will have device available" without mandating they be worn.

We remind educational interpreters (and audiologists, SLPs, and teachers of the Deaf) that the CI does not mean a Deaf student can hear well enough to understand speech (Geers, Tobey, Moog, & Brenner, 2008), and that using ASL does not inhibit a Deaf student with a CI from learning to listen and develop speech skills. This is a complete and utter myth (Mitchell & Karchmer, 2012; Geers, Mitchell, Warner-Czyz, Wang, & Eisenberg, 2017; Pisoni & Cleary, 2004; Knoors & Marschark, 2014).

Boots

As part of a frequency modulation/digital modulation (FM/DM) system, some BTE hearing aids and CIs have a boot/seat plug in attachment. These are designed to have the FM/DM system receiver microphone transmit directly to the hearing aid or CI. Students with an ITE hearing aid will typically wear a neck loop receiver and turn an FM/DM switch on their hearing aid to change it to an infrared receiver. See below for more information on FM/DM systems.

FM/DM Systems

Like interpreting for students who use hearing aids, often educational interpreters are by default responsible for ensuring the classroom FM/DM system is working correctly.

FM and DM systems work in similar ways. The teacher uses a microphone while the Deaf student attaches a receiver to their hearing aid or CI, and the sound is transmitted directly from the microphone to the hearing aid or CI.

Oftentimes, educational interpreters are tasked with checking and changing dead batteries, ensuring the teacher is wearing a microphone, and making sure it is turned on. All educational interpreters should consult with the members of the team and read the FM/DM system manual for troubleshooting.

DC: There are some hilarious narratives of experience from Deaf students whose teachers forgot to turn the microphone off before going to the bathroom or stepping into the hallway for a "private" conversation. Depending on the device range, Deaf students may actually hear things they do not want to.

Flashing Alert Systems

Flashing fire alarms alert Deaf students if there is a fire emergency and are standard requirements in each school building. Deaf students should never be dependent on others to notify them of an emergency.

At home, all Deaf students should have a flashing alert system to notify them of the fire alarm, doorbell, a baby crying, and alarm clocks. If a Deaf student's home is not equipped with these items, it is helpful for an educational interpreter to work with the education team to connect families with appropriate resources.

Videophones

Videophones have fundamentally, and positively, impacted how Deaf people can communicate using technology. Prior to video phones, Deaf people had to rely on a TTY—a teletypewriter-like machine used on regular telephone lines. The TTY is rarely used by Deaf people in modern times—as Deaf people favor the use of videophones.

Any videophone can connect with another videophone, which allows callers to be both seen and heard. For Deaf people, it means they can use signed language to communicate with each other—far less time-consuming than taking turns typing on a TTY. If a Deaf student does not have a videophone at home or on their cell phone, an educational interpreter will want to work with the educational team to provide such resources to the family.

Video Relay Service (VRS)

The ADA (1990) provided for a relay system through the Federal Communications Commission (FCC). This enables Deaf people to communicate with hearing people using a telephone. Historically, this was done using a relay operator and a TTY to "relay" the message to the hearing person on the telephone and vice versa.

With the advent of videophones, Video Relay Service (VRS) provides real-time interpreting services, where the interpreter is at a remote site and an interpreter interprets conversation between a Deaf and a hearing person (Federal Communications Commission, 2023). The Deaf person is on a videophone and the hearing person on a telephone.

Deaf individuals who use spoken language may opt to use a Voice Carryover Service (VCO), which allows the Deaf person to speak over the telephone but receive a text version of what the hearing person is saying.

Video Remote Interpreting (VRI)

Video Remote Interpreting (VRI) is different from VRS. The latter requires the Deaf party to be using a videophone and the hearing party to use a telephone. When using VRS, the parties also cannot be in the same physical location, or it is a violation of FCC rules (Federal Communications Commission, 2023). However, VRI is where an interpreter is interpreting at a distance using a video-based platform (Registry of Interpreters for the Deaf, 2019). This may include a Deaf and a hearing person in the same room with a remote interpreter, or it may include interpreting while no one is in the same physical room such as on a Zoom conference call.

VRI is becoming increasingly popular due to the shortage of interpreters, particularly for emergency situations such as in hospitals when it is difficult to arrange an in-person interpreter in advance (Marsland, Lou, & Snowden, 2010). It is also gaining popularity in schools as an alternative to in-person educational interpreter services, particularly in rural school districts where interpreters may be hard to come by (National Deaf Center on Postsecondary Outcomes, n.d.-b). However, there is no research on the efficacy of VRI in educational settings. Anecdotal data suggest that Deaf students do not attend well to a virtual interpreter, particularly when they are young students without established language.

DC: I did an observation of a middle school student with a VRI interpreter. The student had two laptops—one dedicated for the interpreter and the other for their classwork. They consistently had the VRI interpreter laptop positioned behind their classwork laptop, so they were not able to see the VRI interpreter most of the time.

Captioning

Captions benefit everyone, whether they already have or are developing English language fluency (Hattie, 2012; Szarkowska, Krejtz, Klyszejko, & Wieczorek, 2011). This includes individuals with ADD/ADHD, learning disabilities, English language learners, and more. Additionally, captions can dramatically improve one's ability to retain and recall information from videos. Unlike Deaf students though, hearing viewers can typically keep up with the speed of captioning and primarily use them to augment what they have heard (Szarkowska & Gerber-Morón, 2018).

However, captioning is not a substitute for interpreting. Deaf students cannot rely entirely on captioning as their comprehension is, on average, significantly lower than hearing students' (Cambra, Silvestre, & Leal, 2009; Jelinek Lewis & Jackson, 2001; Marschark et al., 2006). Deaf students will still need an interpretation to be provided.

Closed captions mean the captioning may be turned on or off—as such, educational interpreters should know how to do this on multiple platforms. Open captions are embedded in the video and cannot be turned off. Captioned videos for classroom and educational purposes are available from several national resources, such as the *Described and Captioned Media Program* (Described and Captioned Media Program, n.d.).

It is worth mentioning that auto-captioned materials—captions created by a computer—are not always accurate (VanZant, 2005). Some people even argue no captions are better than poor captions (Kustritz, Rupprecht, & Zhitnitskiy, 2023). Furthermore, since captioning is often 160–200 words per minute (Hattie, 2012), it means that captioned text is very quick and often relies on strong literacy skills to be understood (Cambra, Silvestre, & Leal, 2009; Yoon & Kim, 2011). As such, educational interpreters should continue to interpret all video content regardless of whether or not it is captioned.

SF: I worked with an educational interpreter who would not interpret captioned videos. By the time the Deaf student realized they did not understand the caption, looked at the interpreter, and the interpreter began signing, there was a pronounced delay. Ultimately, the interpretation was not in the spot where the Deaf student was lost, and the video itself was not then accessible. Another educational interpreter would stop interpreting videos when the high school student fell asleep. Everyone notices when the interpreter stops working—thus unintentionally calling out the Deaf student. And while all students should try to stay awake for the video, many hearing students were also napping. Calling the Deaf student out is completely unfair. Bottom line—interpret videos even when the Deaf student has high levels of literacy and/or is sleeping.

Summary

This chapter explored the deep interconnection between culture and interpreting, emphasizing that culture encompasses shared beliefs, values, behaviors, and communication styles. It distinguished between explicit aspects of culture, like food and language, and implicit ones, such as attitudes toward time or space. Interpreters must critically reflect on their own cultural assumptions to provide respectful and effective services. Cultural frameworks—such as monochronic versus polychronic time, individualist versus collectivist orientations, and temporal worldviews—highlight the diversity interpreters must navigate. Language, including ASL, is not just a communication tool but a cultural force that shapes thought and worldview. Cultural identity is layered and intersectional, influenced by race, gender, and disability, making it vital for interpreters to recognize and honor these complexities rather than viewing Deafness in isolation.

Deaf culture is diverse and not monolithic. While many Deaf individuals share values around ASL and visual communication, experiences vary widely based on intersecting identities. Two primary perspectives on Deafness were contrasted: the medical model, which treats Deafness as a deficiency, and the cultural-linguistic model, which affirms Deafness as a valid identity. Educational interpreters, while not inherently part of Deaf culture unless Deaf themselves, serve as cultural stewards who must support Deaf students' access to language, identity, and equitable participation in mainstream environments.

The chapter also delved into ableism, the systemic devaluation of disability, often expressed through seemingly benign behaviors and language that cast disability as something negative. Audism, a specific form of ableism, marginalizes Deaf individuals by prioritizing hearing and speech. Racism intersects with Deaf education, with Black and Indigenous Deaf students facing exclusion and underrepresentation in both educational content and interpreting services. Interpreters are urged to advocate for diversity and representation and to understand the compounding effects of race and Deafness.

Deaf students often find interpreted education less effective than direct instruction due to delays in language access and over-reliance on interpreters as their sole connection to classroom content and peers. They seek autonomy, respect, and interpreters who are knowledgeable and culturally competent. Readiness for interpreting requires a solid language foundation and Theory of Mind, typically developed by third grade. Without these, interpreting may not be effective, and language coaches—Deaf adults who model ASL and foster cognitive development—are recommended.

Language coaches, typically Deaf adults fluent in ASL, provide direct language modeling and support in a natural language environment. They fill the critical gap in language acquisition for Deaf students, particularly those experiencing language deprivation. Coaches focus on building expressive and receptive language skills and cognitive development, preparing students to later benefit from educational interpreters. Coaches differ from interpreters in training and purpose, with a focus on foundational language and identity development.

Deaf interpreters bring unique cultural insight and are especially helpful for students with language deprivation or who are not native ASL users. They work in tandem with hearing interpreters to bridge linguistic and cultural gaps. Deaf students using assistive listening devices such as hearing aids or CIs require tailored support. Although these devices provide auditory access, they do not replace the need for visual language or cultural consideration. Interpreters must understand device functionality and adjust their work accordingly, recognizing that ASL can complement and even enhance spoken language development.

The chapter also addressed the needs of Deaf students with additional disabilities, including DeafBlind students, and those from immigrant or refugee backgrounds. Each group requires specialized strategies, collaboration, and often the inclusion of Deaf interpreters or language coaches. Technology—such as FM/DM systems, captioning, VRS, and VRI—plays a role in access, but it has limitations. Captioning, while useful, is not a substitute for interpreting, and technologies like VRI may not suit all students, especially younger ones. Interpreters must stay informed about accessibility tools and ensure their appropriate use to support full educational access. Overall, cultural competence in educational interpreting demands continuous reflection, learning, and advocacy for inclusive, equitable practices.

Thought Questions

1 How do the changing roles of educational interpreters from elementary school through high school impact Deaf students' independence and social integration? What strategies can educational interpreters use to support, rather than hinder, students' autonomy?
2 How might an interpreter apply the understanding of monochronic vs. polychronic cultural frameworks when working with Deaf students from different backgrounds?
3 What are the effects of systemic discrimination such as ableism and audism on Deaf students? How are these effects compounded by racism for Black, Indigenous, students of color?
4 What are some key indicators that a Deaf student is ready to effectively utilize an educational interpreter?
5 In what ways can language coaches address the challenges of language deprivation among Deaf students? How do their roles differ from those of educational interpreters? How could an educational interpreter incorporate the role of language coaches when working with a Deaf student who has experienced language deprivation?
6 Why is it important for educational interpreters to continue interpreting video content even if it is captioned, and what challenges might arise if they rely solely on captions?

References

Americans with Disabilities Act of 1990, 42 U.S.C. §§ 12101–12213 (2018).

Anderson, K. (2022). Assessing language skills of ASL communicators. Tampa, FL: Supporting Success for Children with Hearing Loss. https://successforkidswithhearingloss.com/wp-content/uploads/2022/02/Assessing-Language-of-ASL-Communicators.pdf.

Antia, S. D., Jones, P. B., Reed, S., & Kreimeyer, K. H. (2009). Academic status and progress of deaf and hard-of-hearing students in general education classrooms. *Journal of Deaf Studies and Deaf Education*, 14(3), 293–311.

ASLized! (2014). The benefits of Deaf interpreters [video]. YouTube. https://www.youtube.com/watch?v=Ec8LjnVuJx8.

Bauman, H.-D. L. (2008). *Open your eyes: Deaf studies talking*. Minneapolis: University of Minnesota Press.

Cambra, C., Silvestre, N., & Leal, A. (2009). Comprehension of television messages by deaf students at various stages of education. *American Annals of the Deaf*, 153(5), 425–434.

Cates, D., & Delkamiller, J. (2021). The impact of sign language interpreter skill on education outcomes in K–12 settings. In E. Winston & S. B. Fitzmaurice (Eds.), *Advances in educational interpreting* (pp. 19–30). Washington, DC: Gallaudet University Press.

Cawthon, S. W., Johnson, P. M., Garberoglio, C. L., & Schoffstall, S. J. (2016). Role models as facilitators of social capital for Deaf individuals: A research synthesis. *American Annals of the Deaf*, 161(2), 115–127.

Center for Atypical Language. (2022a). IEP meeting: Second day [video]. https://vimeo.com/689482372/0f93616a4f.

Center for Atypical Language. (2022b). IEP meeting: Second day: Pre-conference with interpreting team [video]. https://vimeo.com/689369095/11d3826049.

Cerney, B. (2007). Language acquisition, language teaching, and the interpreter as a model for language input. Retrieved from: http://handandmind.org/LgAcquisition.pdf.

Crenshaw, K. W. (1991). Mapping the margins: Intersectionality, identity politics, and violence against women of color. *Stanford Law Review*, 43(6), 1241–1299.

Davis, J. E. (2010). *Hand talk: Sign language among American Indian Nations*. Cambridge: Cambridge University Press.

DeafBlind Interpreting National Training and Resource Center. (n.d.). DeafBlind Interpreting National Training and Resource Center. Western Oregon University. https://www.dbinterpreting.org.

Described and Captioned Media Program (DCMP). (n.d.). About the Described and Captioned Media Program. Silver Spring, MD: National Association of the Deaf.

Dostal, H. M., & Wolbers, K. A. (2014). Developing language and writing skills of deaf and hard of hearing students: A simultaneous approach. *Literacy Research and Instruction*, 53(3), 245–268.

Enns, C. J., Zimmer, K., Boudreault, P., Rabu, S., & Broszeit, C. (2013). *American Sign Language receptive skills test*. Winnipeg, Manitoba: Northern Signs Research.

Farnell, B. M. (1995). *Do you see what I mean? Plains Indian Sign Talk and the embodiment of action*. Austin: University of Texas Press.

Federal Communications Commission (FCC). (2023). Video relay services (VRS). Washington, DC: FCC. https://www.fcc.gov/consumers/guides/video-relay-services.

Fischbeck, N. (2021). Educational interpreters' strategies to support Deaf refugee and immigrant students. In E. A. Winston & S. B. Fitzmaurice (Eds.), *Advances in educational interpreting* (pp. 123–145). Washington, DC: Gallaudet University Press.

Fitzmaurice, S. (2021). The realistic role metaphor for educational interpreters. In E. A. Winston & S. B. Fitzmaurice (Eds.), *Advances in educational interpreting* (pp. 285–307). Washington, DC: Gallaudet University Press.

Fitzmaurice, S. (2024). Food for thought: Terms matter. *VIEWS*, 41(4), 24–25.

Gagnon, E. B., Eskridge, H., Brown, K. D., & Park, L. R. (2021). The impact of cumulative cochlear implant wear time on spoken language outcomes at age 3 years. *Journal of Speech, Language, and Hearing Research*, 64(4), 1369–1375.

Geers, A. E., Mitchell, C. M., Warner-Czyz, A., Wang, N. Y., & Eisenberg, L. S. (2017). Early sign language exposure and cochlear implantation benefits. *Pediatrics*, 140(1), e20163489.

Geers, A. E., Tobey, E. A., Moog, J. S., & Brenner, C. (2008). Long-term outcomes of cochlear implantation in the preschool years: From elementary grades to high school. *International Journal of Audiology*, 47(Suppl 2), S21–S30.

Goss, B. (2003). Hearing from the deaf culture. *Intercultural Communication Studies*, 12 (2), 1–17.

Guardino, C. (2015). Evaluating teachers' preparedness to work with students who are deaf and hard of hearing with disabilities. *American Annals of the Deaf*, 160(4), 415–426.

Hall, E. T. (1976). *Beyond culture*. Garden City, NY: Anchor Press/Doubleday.

Hall, E. T. (1983). *The dance of life: The other dimension of time*. Garden City, NY: Anchor Press/Doubleday.

Hall-Katter, J., Leffler, L., & Perez, J. (2020). Center for Deaf and Hard of Hearing Education ASL Skills Checklist (revised June 2022). Indiana Department of Health, Center for Deaf and Hard of Hearing Education. https://www.in.gov/health/cdhhe/files/Center-ASL-Skills-Checklist-June-2022.pdf.

Hands & Voices. (n.d.). Self-advocacy and use of an educational interpreter. Hands & Voices. https://www.handsandvoices.org/articles/education/advocacy/V9-3_selfAdvocacy.htm.

Hattie, J. (2012). *Visible learning for teachers: Maximizing impact on learning*. London: Routledge.

Hauser, P. C., O'Hearn, A., McKee, M., Steider, A., & Thew, D. (2010). Deaf epistemology: Deafhood and Deafness. *American Annals of the Deaf*, 154(5), 486–492.

Hofstede, G. (2001). *Culture's consequences: Comparing values, behaviors, institutions, and organizations across nations* (2nd ed.). Thousand Oaks, CA: Sage Publications.

Holcomb, T. K., & Smith, D. H. (Eds.) (2018). *Deaf eyes on interpreting*. Washington, DC: Gallaudet University Press.

Hoover, W. A., & Gough, P. B. (1990). The simple view of reading. *Reading and Writing*, 2(2), 127–160.

Hopper, M. J. (2025). Incidental learning with deaf students. *Journal of Deaf Studies and Deaf Education*, 30(2), 286–288.

Jelinek Lewis, M. S., & Jackson, D. W. (2001). Television literacy: Comprehension of program content using closed captions for the deaf. *Journal of Deaf Studies and Deaf Education*, 6(1), 43–53.

Johnson, R. E., Liddell, S. K., & Erting, C. J. (1994). *Unlocking the curriculum: Principles for achieving access in Deaf education*. Washington, DC: Gallaudet Research Institute, Gallaudet University.

Kendon, A. (1988). *Sign languages of Aboriginal Australia: Cultural, semiotic and communicative perspectives*. Cambridge: Cambridge University Press.

Klima, E. S., & Bellugi, U. (1979). *The signs of language*. Cambridge, MA: Harvard University Press.

Knoors, H., & Marschark, M. (2014). *Teaching deaf learners: Psychological and developmental foundations*. New York: Oxford University Press.

Kurz, K. B. (2023). Deaf interpreters as educational interpreters. In L. J. Johnson, M. M. Taylor, B. Schick, S. E. Brown, L. Bolster, & E. G. Girardin (Eds.), *Complexities in educational interpreting: An investigation into patterns of practice* (pp. 19–21). Edmonton: Interpreting Consolidated.

Kurz, K. B., & Langer, E. C. (2004). Student perspectives on educational interpreting: Twenty deaf and hard of hearing students offer insights and suggestions. In E. A. Winston (Ed.), *Educational interpreting: How it can succeed* (pp. 9–40). Washington, DC: Gallaudet University Press.

Kurz, K. B., Schick, B., & Hauser, P. C. (2015). Deaf children's science content learning in direct instruction versus interpreted instruction. *Journal of Science Education for Students with Disabilities*, 18(1), 23–37.

Kustritz, M., Rupprecht, R, & Zhitnitskiy, P. (2023). Comparison of accuracy of machine-generated or human-generated captions of Zoom live lectures in a comparative theriogenology course. *Clinical Theriogenology*, 15, 9596.

LaBue, M. A. (1998). *Interpreted education: A study of deaf students' access to the content and form of literacy instruction in a mainstreamed high school English class* (Unpublished doctoral dissertation). Harvard University.

Ladd, P. (2003). *Understanding Deaf culture: In search of Deafhood.* Clevedon: Multilingual Matters.

Lane, H., Hoffmeister, R., & Bahan, B. (1996). *A journey into the Deaf-World.* San Diego, CA: DawnSignPress.

Lederberg, A. R., Schick, B., & Spencer, P. E. (2013). Language and literacy development of deaf and hard-of-hearing children: Successes and challenges. *Developmental Psychology*, 49(1), 15–30.

Leigh, I. W., Andrews, J. F., & Harris, R. L. (2016). *Deaf culture: Exploring deaf communities in the United States* (2nd ed.). San Diego, CA: Plural Publishing.

Lucy, A. (2001). Sapir–Whorf hypothesis. In N. J. Smelser & P. B. Baltes (Eds.), *International encyclopedia of the social & behavioral sciences* (pp. 903–906). Oxford: Pergamon.

Marschark, M., Leigh, G., Sapere, P., Burnham, D., Convertino, C., Stinson, M., Knoors, H., Vervloed, M., & Noble, W. (2006). Benefits of sign language interpreting and text alternatives for deaf students' classroom learning. *Journal of Deaf Studies and Deaf Education*, 11(4), 421–437.

Marschark, M., Sapere, P., Convertino, C. M., & Pelz, J. (2008). Learning via direct and mediated instruction by deaf students. *Journal of Deaf Studies and Deaf Education*, 13 (4), 546–561.

Marschark, M., & Knoors, H. (2015). *Educating deaf learners: Creating a global evidence base.* New York: Oxford University Press.

Marsland, M. C., Lou, C., & Snowden, L. (2010). Use of communication technologies to cost-effectively increase the availability of interpretation services in healthcare settings. *Telemedicine Journal of E-Health*, 16(6), 739–745.

McCaskill, C., Lucas, C., Bayley, R., & Hill, J. C. (2011). *The hidden treasure of black ASL: Its history and structure.* Washington, DC: Gallaudet University Press.

McCray, C. L. (2013). *A phenomenological study of the relationship between deaf students in higher education and their sign language interpreters* (Unpublished Dissertation). UMI Number: 3576030.

Miner, C. (2021). Interpreting for deaf and hard of hearing emergent signers in academia. In E. A. Winston & S. B. Fitzmaurice (Eds.), *Advances in educational interpreting* (pp. 68–108). Washington, DC: Gallaudet University Press.

Mitchell, R. E., & Karchmer, M. A. (2012). Demographics and achievement characteristics of deaf and hard of hearing students. In M. Marschark & P. E. Spencer (Eds.),

The Oxford handbook of deaf studies, language, and education (2nd ed., pp. 18–31). New York: Oxford University Press.

Mowry, R. L. (1994). What deaf high school seniors tell us about their social networks. In C. J. Erting, R. C. Johnson, D. L. Smith, & B. D. Snider (Eds.), *The deaf way: Perspectives from the international conference on deaf culture* (pp. 642–649). Washington, DC: Gallaudet University Press.

Mukari, S. Z., Ling, L. N., & Ghani, H. A. (2007). Educational performance of pediatric cochlear implant recipients in mainstream classes. *International Journal of Pediatric Otorhinolaryngology*, 71(2), 231–240.

Musselman, C., Mootilal, A., & MacKay, S. (1996). The social adjustment of deaf adolescents in segregated, partially integrated, and mainstreamed settings. *Journal of Deaf Studies and Deaf Education*, 1(1), 52–63.

Nash, J. C. (2008). Re-thinking intersectionality. *Feminist Review*, 89(1), 1–15.

National Deaf Center on Postsecondary Outcomes. (n.d.-a). Shira's story: Role of interpreters. National Deaf Center. https://nationaldeafcenter.org/resource-items/shiras-story-role-of-interpreters/.

National Deaf Center on Postsecondary Outcomes. (n.d.-b). Remote interpreting services. National Deaf Center. https://www.nationaldeafcenter.org/resources/access-accommodations/coordinating-services/interpreting/video-remote-interpreting/.

Nuccio, J., & Clark, J. L. (2020). Protactile linguistics: Discussing recent research findings. *Journal of American Sign Languages and Literatures*, 5(2), 45–60.

Oliva, G. A., & Risser Lytle, L. (2014). *Turning the tide: Making life better for deaf and hard of hearing schoolchildren*. Washington, DC: Gallaudet University Press.

Padden, C., & Humphries, T. (1988). *Deaf in America: Voices from a culture*. Cambridge, MA: Harvard University Press.

Paul, P. V. (Ed.) (2020). *The education of d/Deaf and hard of hearing children: Perspectives on language and literacy development*. Basel: Education Sciences/MDPI.

Peterson, R., & Monikowski, C. (2010). Perceptions of efficacy of sign language interpreters working in K-12 settings. In K. M. Christensen (Ed.), *Ethical considerations in educating children who are deaf or hard of hearing* (pp. 129–153). Washington, DC: Gallaudet University Press.

Pisoni, D. B., & Cleary, M. (2004). Learning, memory, and cognitive processes in deaf children following cochlear implantation. In F.-G. Zeng, A. N. Popper, & R. R. Fay (Eds.), *Cochlear implants: Auditory prostheses and electric hearing* (pp. 377–426). New York: Springer.

Prinzi, L. M. (2023). Deaf student–interpreter relationships and feedback practices in K-12 mainstream deaf education. *Journal of Deaf Studies and Deaf Education*, 28(1), 68–83.

Registry of Interpreters for the Deaf (RID). (2018). *Annual report*. Alexandria, VA: RID. https://rid.org/programs/membership/publications/.

Registry of Interpreters for the Deaf (RID). (2019). Standard practice paper: Video remote interpreting (VRI). Alexandria, VA: RID. https://rid.org/resources/#spp.

Russell, D. (2008). What do others think of our work? Deaf students, teachers, administrators, and parent perspectives on educational interpreting. In C. Roy (Ed.), *Diversity and community in the worldwide sign language interpreting profession: Proceedings of the 2nd WASLI Conference* (pp. 34–38). Coleford: Douglas McLean Publishing.

Russell, D., & McLeod, J. (2009). Educational interpreting: Multiple perspectives of our work. In J. Mole (Ed.), *International perspectives on educational interpreting* (pp. 128–144). Brassington: Direct Learn Services Ltd.

Schick, B. (2004). How might learning through an educational interpreter influence cognitive development? In E. A. Winston (Ed.), *Educational interpreting: How it can succeed* (pp. 73–87). Washington, DC: Gallaudet University Press.

Schick, B. (2008). A model of learning within an interpreted K–12 educational setting. In M. Marschark & P. Hauser (Eds.), *Deaf cognition: Foundations and outcomes* (pp. 351–386). New York: Oxford University Press.

Schick, B., Williams, K., & Kupermintz, H. (2006). Look who's being left behind: Educational interpreters and access to education for deaf and hard-of-hearing students. *Journal of Deaf Studies and Deaf Education*, 11(1), 3–20.

Simms, L., Baker, S., & Clark, M. D. (2013). The standardized visual communication and sign language checklist for signing children. *Sign Language Studies*, 14(1), 101–124.

Singer, S. J., Cacciato, K., Kamenakis, J., & Shapiro, A. (2020). Determining language and inclusion for Deaf-Plus children. *International Electronic Journal of Elementary Education*, 13(1), 1–19.

Stewart, M. (2020, October 16). Deaf and hard of hearing community suffers from dearth of diverse interpreters. Insight Into Diversity. https://www.insightintodiversity.com/deaf-and-hard-of-hearing-community-suffers-from-dearth-of-diverse-interpreters/.

Szarkowska, A., & Gerber-Morón, O. (2018). Viewers can keep up with fast subtitles: Evidence from eye movements. *PLoS ONE*, 13(6), 1–30.

Szarkowska, A., Krejtz, I., Klyszejko, Z., & Wieczorek, A. (2011). Verbatim, standard, or edited?: Reading patterns of different captioning styles among deaf, hard of hearing, and hearing viewers. *American Annals of the Deaf*, 156(4), 363–378.

The Diversity Academy. (2025). The Diversity Academy. https://www.thediversityacademy.com.

Thibodeau, R. (2021). A native-user approach: The value of certified deaf interpreters in K-12 settings. In E. A. Winston & S. B. Fitzmaurice (Eds.), *Advances in educational interpreting* (pp. 31–43). Washington, DC: Gallaudet University Press.

Triandis, H. C. (1995). *Individualism & collectivism*. Boulder, CO: Westview Press.

United States Government Accountability Office (GAO). (2018). *K–12 education: Discipline disparities for Black students, boys, and students with disabilities* (GAO-18-258). Washington, DC: GAO. https://www.gao.gov/assets/gao-18-258.pdf.

VanZant, M. (2005). *An analysis of real-time captioning errors: Implications for teachers* (Unpublished Master's Thesis). Rochester Institute of Technology. https://repository.rit.edu/theses/4024/.

Watkins, S., Pittman, P., & Walden, B. (1998). The deaf mentor experimental project for young children who are deaf and their families. *American Annals of the Deaf*, 143(1), 29–34.

Wie, O. B., von Koss Torkildsen, J., Schauber, S., Busch, T., & Litovsky, R. (2020). Long-term language development in children with early simultaneous bilateral cochlear implants. *Ear and Hearing*, 41(5), 1294–1305.

Winston, E. A. (1985). Mainstreaming: Like it or not. *Journal of Interpretation*, 2, 117–119.

Winston, E. A. (1990). Mainstream interpreting: An analysis of the task. In L. Swabey (Ed.), *Proceedings of the eighth national convention of the Conference of Interpreter Trainers* (pp. 51–67). Pomona, CA: CIT Publications.

Winston, E. A. (1994). An interpreted education: Inclusion or exclusion? In R. C. Johnson and O. P. Cohen (Eds.), *Implications and complications for deaf students of the full inclusion movement* (pp. 55–62). Gallaudet Research Institute Occasional Paper 94–2. Washington, DC: Gallaudet Research Institute.

Wolters, N., Knoors, H., Cillessen, A. H., & Verhoeven, L. (2012). Impact of peer and teacher relations on deaf early adolescents' well-being: Comparisons before and after a major school transition. *Journal of Deaf Studies and Deaf Education*, 17(4), 463–482.

Yoon, J. O., & Kim, M. (2011). The effects of captions on deaf students' content comprehension, cognitive load, and motivation in online learning. *American Annals of the Deaf*, 156(3), 283–289.

Zeshan, U., & de Vos, C. (Eds.). (2012). *Sign languages in village communities: Anthropological and linguistic insights*. Berlin: De Gruyter Mouton.

6 Language and Literacy

Understanding the distinctions between language, modality, and communication is essential for anyone working in Deaf education, particularly educational interpreters. Language is not merely a tool for expression; it is a structured, rule-governed system that underpins cognitive development, social interaction, and academic success. Modality refers to the sensory means—spoken, signed, or written—through which language is conveyed, whereas communication encompasses all methods of transmitting meaning, both linguistic and non-linguistic. For Deaf children, access to a natural, fully accessible language like American Sign Language (ASL) during the critical period of early childhood is a prerequisite for healthy cognitive, social, and linguistic development. This chapter explores the consequences of language deprivation, including its impact on Theory of Mind and literacy acquisition, and highlights the crucial role educational interpreters play in supporting Deaf students. By making informed, strategic language choices, interpreters help bridge the gap between ASL and English, fostering deeper comprehension and lifelong learning.

Language Development

The terms *language, modality*, and *communication* are frequently used in educational settings, and it is important to understand the differences between these three terms. Oftentimes, the focus with Deaf children is on communication and not on language. However, a growing body of research on language deprivation points to a need to consider language, not just communication, for Deaf children (Cerney, 2007; Friedmann & Rusou, 2015; Hall, Hall, & Caselli, 2019; Johnson, Liddell, & Erting, 1989; Knoors & Marschark, 2014; Langer & Schick, 2004; Marschark & Hauser, 2012; Marschark & Knoors, 2012; Marschark & Wauters, 2008; Mayberry, 2002; Mayberry & Locke, 2003; Morford & Mayberry, 2000; Mounty, Pucci, & Harmon, 2013; Petitto et al., 2001).

A language is a complex, rule-governed system capable of conveying abstract thought. For a system to be considered a language, it must have arbitrariness, cultural transmission, discreteness, duality, productivity, and displacement (Fromkin, Rodman, & Hyams, 2018; Valli, Lucas, Mulrooney, & Villanueva, 2011). Arbitrariness means there is not a transparent relationship between the

DOI: 10.4324/9781003423058-6

word and the concept it references (i.e., nothing about the English word "cat" corresponds to the furry four-legged monster that pukes in your shoes). Signed languages have substantially more iconicity than spoken languages, but there are still many lexical signs and grammatical elements that are arbitrary (Meier, 2002). Cultural transmission means that language is passed down from person to person within a family or culture. Discreteness means that there is a meaningful distinction between the phonemes of a language. In spoken languages, phonemes are the individual sounds that exist in that language, and a small number of sounds can be recombined into an infinite number of words (Yule, 2020). In signed languages, there are individual handshapes, palm orientations, movements, and locations, and a small set of each can be recombined into an infinite number of signs. That is the property of duality—individual phonemes do not mean anything, but when combined with other phonemes, you get something meaningful. Productivity means that human languages have the capacity for infinite creation of unique utterances (Fromkin, Rodman, & Hyams, 2018). Many sentences in this book are words arranged in ways in which they never have been before. The property of displacement means language can be used to refer to things not in the immediate environment. Displacement allows humans to talk about phenomena of eons past, and to plan for the future.

Modality is how language or communication is expressed (i.e., signed, spoken, written, etc.) or received (i.e., visual, auditory, tactile). We include touch for receptive language because Braille and tactile forms of signed languages are received via touch. Tactile modalities are important for the education of DeafBlind students. The acronym "LSL"—meaning listening and spoken language—has come into prevalence in the past couple of decades as the oralist/manualist debate has heated up in the wake of the LEAD-K movement (LEAD-K, n.d.). See how the terms "listening" and "spoken" refer to modality and not language? This kind of error is incredibly common, so be sure that when talking about language you are using the names of languages instead of modalities.

Communication is the act of conveying your intentions to another. Communication can occur without language (Owens, 2016). Think of a young child who needs to go to the bathroom doing the well-known "potty dance." Even though the child may be saying nothing to you via language, the movements of their body communicate clearly to you they need to go to the bathroom. Crying, kicking, hitting, running, pointing, and laughing are all forms of communication. When Individualized Education Program (IEP) Teams focus on a child's communication rather than their language, they are neglecting a critical part of cognitive development for which communication systems are not a substitute.

Language Acquisition

Language acquisition proceeds in stages. These stages occur in order in the development of any language in any modality. The first stage of language acquisition involves responding to affect (the emotion expressed in a person's face or voice), responding to one's own name, understanding common words, communicating differently with pre-verbal smiles or cries, pointing to objects to express wants and needs, babbling, making eye contact, and initiating interaction with adults (Friedmann & Rusou, 2015). In typical language acquisition, these all occur within the first year of life.

The second broad stage of language acquisition occurs late in the first year of life and into the second. This includes concentrating on most things in the environment, being distracted by language in the environment, answering simple WH- questions, understanding more language than is produced, understanding that things have names, using words to communicate, and making up words (Hoff, 2013). Incidentally, many Deaf students have goals in their IEPs to work with a speech language pathologist or teacher of the Deaf on answering WH- questions. This is a hallmark of language deprivation.

More advanced language acquisition occurs between two and three years of age in typical language acquisition. Here, toddlers can enjoy rhythmic patterns in language, understand verbs and instructions using them, put two or more words together, and use a variety of word types (Owens, 2016). Incidentally, increasing *mean length of utterance* is another common IEP goal area for Deaf students.

Regardless of the age someone is when they are first exposed to language, acquisition proceeds in this order. For humans, the critical period for language acquisition is within the first five years of life, meaning any human with typical neural development will acquire any language that is consistently accessible to them in their environment (Lenneberg, 1967). If a child is regularly exposed to multiple accessible languages during this critical period, they will acquire multiple languages. The brain is sensitive to language in the environment during this time, but it does not seem to be sensitive to the specific modality of the language (Mayberry, 2007). Therefore, a child can learn signed or spoken languages with equivalent ease in those early years. Think about children of Deaf adults (CODAs). They are hearing children of Deaf adults who acquire a signed language as their first language while at the same time acquiring spoken language used in the environment around them.

As CODAs are able to acquire a spoken and a signed language simultaneously, so can other children, including Deaf children. However, there is still a persistent belief in the medical community that Deaf children need to focus on spoken language acquisition first and then work on developing a signed language later in life if spoken language acquisition fails (National Association of the Deaf, n.d.). Parents are often counseled by the doctors and audiologists they encounter early in their Deaf child's life to use auditory/aural approaches (Hall, Hall, & Caselli, 2019). Remember—auditory and aural are modalities, not languages. This advice frequently results in language deprivation.

Language Deprivation

Many Deaf children struggle with learning language during their school years, due to having minimal language competence in either English or ASL (or their home language). This factor alone is a significant hurdle because the prime window of language acquisition is birth to age five. By the time children start school, this window is already closing.

Language deprivation is due to a chronic lack of full access to a natural language during the prime window of language acquisition, also called the "critical period." The longer a child's access to language is delayed, the more severe, pervasive, and lasting the effects are on their cognitive development (Cheng, Roth, Halgren, & Mayberry, 2019). This is referred to as *Language Deprivation Syndrome*.

Language Deprivation Syndrome symptoms include a lack of understanding of basic abstract concepts, an inability to arrange a narrative in sequential order, difficulty with working memory, an inability to organize facts into cause and effect relationships, an inability to explain why or how things happen, ease in acquiring nouns but difficulty with acquiring verbs or adjectives, a lack of ordinary grammatical features in language, a lack of awareness of the conversational partners' need for context (Theory of Mind), and severe deficits in personal and world knowledge (Gulati, 2019; Hall, 2017). These all occur in the known absence of accessible language early in a child's life.

Children with Language Deprivation Syndrome exhibit communicative intent and produce vocabulary accurately (Hall, Levin, & Anderson, 2017). Deaf children commonly have goals on their IEPs related to answering WH- questions, sequentially arranging stories, and learning abstract concepts. If you work with a child with any of these specified as goals in their IEP, that is a pretty decent indication that the child has language deprivation and that knowledge will heavily influence how you interpret.

Without addressing those language deficits, there are long-term consequences for reading comprehension, mental health, social development, and cognitive development. Caselli, Hall, and Henner (2020) write, "Deafness affects the way that language is transmitted, while language deprivation affects the entire linguistic system" (p. 1329).

Language acquisition also occurs in context. When you acquire language as an infant, you acquire it because languages used around you are connected to experiences you are having. Think about when an adult speaks to a child about a dog. They may say, "Oh, look at the doggie! Let's pet the doggie. Look at the nice doggie." During such an interaction, the child hears the word "doggie" repeatedly while actually having a dog there in front of them. This helps them to make the connection between that cluster of sounds and the object in front of them. The same thing happens with sign language acquisition when an adult points to an object and then gives the object's name while in the child's line of sight.

Language acquisition requires significant interaction and direct communication in context, and interpreters are typically trained to work with clients who have at least one fully functional (native) language. Interpreters are not trained to work with clients who do not have a native language. For educational interpreters, this means that if a Deaf student has a native language, then they have the ability to connect the language they know with the language they are learning in school, and educational interpreter services are more likely to be an appropriate accommodation. Without a foundational language upon which to build, a Deaf student cannot benefit from an educational interpreter who is functioning as "just" an interpreter (i.e., if the interpreter is just taking information from one language and interpreting it into the other language without adding any context, background information, vocabulary instruction, or other supports). Educational interpreters cannot serve as language models for a Deaf child's first language acquisition while also interpreting, as the input is not interactional and is at best incomplete (Marschark, Sapere, Convertino, & Seewagen, 2005; Peterson & Monikowski, 2010; Schick, 2004; 2008).

The best remedy for Language Deprivation Syndrome is for the student to work with a language coach (see chapter five). However, if as an educational interpreter you work with a child with language deprivation, one of the only things you can do as an interpreter is to provide materials, pictures, videos, and use things in the environment to give context to the words that you are signing. Standing in front of the classroom and interpreting about whatever the teacher is talking about will not be effective for a child with language deprivation. Such students need more context given to everything that is signed to them to make connections between the world and the abstract symbols of language.

Cognitive Development and Theory of Mind

Unfortunately, often due to language deprivation and delays, Deaf children experience delays in cognitive development (Schick, 2004). Whether one needs language to develop cognitively or whether one can only have their cognitive abilities assessed with language is a moot point for our work as educational interpreters. We know executive functioning such as planning and organizing can also be delayed because of language deprivation (Courtin, Melot, & Corroyer, 2008; Hauser, Lukomski, & Hillman, 2008). Adding to that, simply using an interpreter adds a cognitive workload as we have pointed out in previous sections.

Theory of Mind is a cognitive skill that refers to the ability to understand that other people have thoughts, wants, beliefs, desires, intentions, and perspectives that differ from our own (Schick, de Villiers, de Villiers, & Hoffmeister, 2007). Theory of Mind skills are a critical ingredient for social interaction, empathy, communication, and conflict resolution because they enable people to predict and interpret the behavior of others.

Generally, by age three, children begin to recognize others have different desires and, by age five, can understand that others' beliefs can be false. Beyond that, Theory of Mind skills continue to develop as children begin to comprehend more complex mental states and intentions (Wellman & Liu, 2004). An absence of Theory of Mind skills inhibits how we interact with and understand people around us.

Deaf children score significantly below hearing peers on Theory of Mind tasks (Peterson & Slaughter, 2006). However, Deaf children who acquire language before age ten are more likely to develop sufficient Theory of Mind skills. And those Deaf children with age-appropriate language development skills usually perform better than those children with language deficits (Marschark & Hauser, 2008; Hale & Tager-Flusberg, 2003). However, those cognitive skills are still frequently below those of hearing peers simply because Deaf children cannot benefit as much from incidental learning as hearing children. There is ample evidence that using a cochlear implant does not benefit a Deaf student's development of Theory of Mind skills. At its most basic level, how can you describe what someone else is feeling without any language skills?

Literacy Development

We circle back to the implications of language deprivation in terms of literacy development. Language deprivation sets a Deaf child up for a lifetime of stifled language abilities, which thereby affect their literacy development (Humphries et al., 2012; Marschark & Spencer, 2009).

One of the fundamental goals of the educational system is to develop literacy. However, the development of literacy skills requires a language foundation—that is, you must have a language before you can connect print to meaning. In other words, literacy in a second language (aka English for Deaf students) is directly supported by the Deaf student's foundation in ASL. Students with a strong foundation in ASL can develop literacy at the same pace as hearing peers (Allen, Letteri, Choi, & Dang, 2014; Snoddon, Small, & Cripps, 2004). As an educational interpreter, you will experience interpreting for language arts instruction at every grade level, as English is the only core subject matter required across all 12 grades.

Unfortunately, schools are not designed to teach a child their first language but, as we have discussed, many Deaf children are language deprived and so start their educational program without a fully functional first language. However, one of the prerequisites for learning to read is an extant language.

The most straightforward model of how we learn to read is called the *Simple View of Reading* (SVR), which promotes the idea that your ability to recognize words, combined with your ability to comprehend language, is what results in your ability to comprehend what you read (Gough & Tunmer, 1986; Hoover & Gough, 1990). The SVR indicates the ability to recognize words involves phonological awareness, phonics, and word fluency. Language comprehension involves the comprehension of vocabulary, language, concepts, and ability to communicate (Snow, 2002). A common conceptualization of the SVR is Scarborough's Reading Rope (McCardle, Scarborough, & Catts, 2001). The upper strand is language comprehension which includes background knowledge, vocabulary, language structures, verbal reasoning, and literacy knowledge. The lower strand is word recognition and encompasses phonological awareness, decoding, and sight recognition. The upper strand skills become increasingly strategic in reading and the lower strands become increasingly automatic. Once these strands have woven together, you have skilled reading with comprehension. Literacy interventions often focus on one or more of these strands.

Much like with language acquisition, print literacy has different stages of development. As an individual learns how to read, their ability to manipulate and develop units of print grows in complexity. A hot topic in literacy instruction is the *science of reading*, which has five foundational principles that support the development of reading comprehension in hearing children with an established first language (National Institute of Child Health and Human Development, 2000). These include phonological awareness, phonics and word recognition, fluency, vocabulary and oral language comprehension, and text comprehension. The science of reading is the components of the SVR broken down into instructional areas. Each area is addressed below.

Phonological Awareness

Phonological awareness is the ability to recognize and manipulate the smallest unit of a language. In spoken languages, these are the sounds in words. Signed languages do not have sounds, but they do have a phonological level. You may have learned in your ASL classes about handshape, location, palm orientation, and movement. These are considered the building blocks of signed languages, the same way spoken languages have sounds as their building blocks. These building blocks are called *phonemes*—they are meaningless on their own, but meaningful when used in combination (Yule, 2020).

There are many more possible handshapes, locations, movements, and palm orientations than are used in any given signed language. The same is true for sounds in spoken languages. The human mouth can create many more sounds than you will hear distinguished in any one spoken language. To see all possible phonemes in spoken languages, look up the International Phonetic Alphabet (International Phonetic Association, 1999). Each spoken language has its own unique subset of these phonemes.

How you identify that a language has a certain phoneme is by testing for minimal pairs—finding two words that differ only based on that one sound (in a spoken language) or parameter (in a signed language). An example of a minimal pair in English would be the words *pat* and *bat*; by changing the first sound, you get a different word. This tells you that */p/* and */b/* are phonemes in English. An example in ASL would be the signs FATHER and MOTHER. The only thing that changes about the articulation of those two signs is the location—FATHER is signed on the forehead and MOTHER is signed on the chin. Therefore, you know that the forehead and the chin are two distinct locations in ASL because you can find signs whose meaning is different just by changing the location to the forehead or the chin. Since both English and ASL have phonemes, it is possible to have phonological awareness in both English and ASL.

As an educational interpreter, you will need to understand how phoneme manipulation works in both languages in order to be able to interpret in a linguistically and culturally equivalent way. When Deaf students are developing their foundational literacy skills, the ability to understand, identify, and manipulate the phonemes in their signed language correlates with their ability to do the same with alphabetic print (Mayberry, del Giudice, & Lieberman, 2011; McQuarrie & Abbott, 2013; Morford & Carlson, 2011).

Phonics

Phonics has to do with understanding sound-spelling patterns between words in their spoken form and words in their written form (National Institute of Child Health and Human Development, 2000). When someone writes a word *phonetically*, they are spelling it out using the rules of sound–letter mapping, which may or may not match the actual spelling of the word. Whereas some print languages like Spanish have a one-to-one mapping of letters to sounds, English does not. Think about the letter cluster *-ough*. It can be pronounced several different ways, as in the words: thought, though, rough, through, and bough. Phonetically, these words would be spelled: thot, tho, ruf, throo, and bow. Therefore, some words must be learned as a whole unit, because applying the rules of phonics would lead to an inaccurate pronunciation or spelling.

Phonics is a big deal in reading instruction because the assumption is that you already speak the language, so accessing the meaning of a word from print just requires you to sound it out (Snow, 2002). Once you sound it out, you match it to the sound pattern of a word you already know. At that point, you have "read" the word. The assumption is that children starting school have a spoken language vocabulary of roughly 3,500 words, so learning to read is a matter of matching print words to that vocabulary. From there, students learn strategies to puzzle out the meanings of new words that they have not heard before.

However, Deaf children do not have the same spoken English vocabularies as their peers when they start school. If they experience language deprivation, their vocabularies will be smaller. If they have access to a signed language from birth, then their vocabulary will be signed, not spoken. The bottom line is phonics does not work to support Deaf children's ability to decode print. Bilingual instructional approaches for Deaf children use more of a whole-word approach to early literacy, where children learn to recognize whole printed words matched with signed concepts instead of sound patterns (Mounty, Pucci, & Harmon, 2013).

Word Fluency

Word fluency is related to a person's ability to rapidly and accurately identify words in a text (Snow, 2002). When children learn to read, they start with letter sounds, then learn to blend sounds to read words. As children identify the sound pattern that matches what they have read, they can then access the meaning that they have stored in their brain. That process takes quite a bit of time in early literacy development.

As children become more fluent readers, they have more *automatic word recognition*—that is, the ability to very rapidly identify a word without having to sound out every single letter of every single word (Ehri, 2005). As they develop more automatic word recognition, their overall reading fluency increases. However, it is possible to have *oral fluency* in reading without using a spoken language if they can rapidly identify, understand, and integrate the meanings of the words they are reading.

As an educational interpreter, you will experience working with Deaf children who have been taught to decode print without necessarily encoding meaning from it—that is, it *looks like they can read*, but they cannot answer any comprehension questions about what they have read. For Deaf children using spoken English expressively, they are often able to pronounce their way through sentences without having any idea what they mean (Marschark & Hauser, 2008). Some Deaf children will have a mix of spoken English and ASL, or a manual communication system, and have learned a sign for each word so that they can sign through sentences without knowing what they mean.

Word fluency is tested for speed—how many words you can read in one minute minus errors you make. These tests do not account for comprehension, just speed. To make matters worse, one of the ways teachers boost reading fluency is with sight words. These are high-frequency words in English print, or words that do not have a clear sound–letter mapping. Unfortunately, many of these words are part of English grammar but have little substantial meaning, such as *the, is, are, at, am, an*. As an educational interpreter, you will need to constantly gauge how much the Deaf student comprehends what they are reading, especially in early elementary grades when children are still learning to read. See the section in chapter four on interpreting English language arts classes for more suggestions and considerations.

Vocabulary Comprehension

Vocabulary comprehension involves not just understanding what words mean but also understanding how they are used (Beck & McKeown, 2007). Words do not exist in isolation in our brains. Since words are learned in context, we store words with their context, such that a single word can bring to mind a whole host of experiences, including related words. This is called our semantic network (Collins & Quillian, 1969). When you see or hear a word, you access everything around that word that your knowledge and your experience provide you. Deaf children often have very shallow semantic depth. What this means is that they rarely have multiple definitions for words, and do not make connections between a word that they see and their experiences surrounding the concept it represents.

Language instruction must be deliberate, but too often the necessary context is missing because literacy instruction is *designed* for children who already know about words in context. Manual communication systems used in Deaf Education (discussed later in this chapter) rarely consider conceptual accuracy, so Deaf children may learn one sign for one English word even though that English word may have many meanings.

Hearing children acquire different meanings of words through incidental learning—just hearing the word used in different contexts builds an understanding of multiple meanings. Deaf children miss out on this, especially if they are made to use only a spoken language outside of school.

This broader understanding of the world, this extra linguistic knowledge, this ability to reason with language, is one of the things that is lost in language deprivation. This results in lasting difficulties with becoming a skilled, fluent reader. Therefore, it is no small task for educational interpreters to interpret for Deaf children during language arts time. Educational interpreters must constantly assess what the child knows, what they have names for, and how they are understanding how words fit together.

Often, early measures of literacy skill have to do with reading fluency, so the focus is often on getting Deaf students either to pronounce words quickly, or to be able to quickly decode into signs words that they see in print. As an educational interpreter, one of your responsibilities is to gauge what the student is comprehending of what they are reading and inform IEP Team members when you suspect that a child can sign their way through a list of words or a list of sentences without comprehension.

Text Comprehension

Text-level comprehension is the goal of any literacy instruction (National Institute of Child Health and Human Development, 2000). It is the ability to take a series of phrases and sentences and to make sense of what they mean. When working with Deaf children in educational settings, this is an area where educational interpreters will often see students struggle. Many factors contribute to difficulty with text-level comprehension, but language deprivation is a big one for Deaf children.

Text comprehension requires children to have a large vocabulary in the first place, but it also requires them to understand how words are used in different contexts and by different people. Often, people who are learning another language struggle with idiomatic language, or any phrases where the whole is not readily apparent from the individual meanings of the words (Kecskes, 2015). Think of the phrase "people who live in glass houses shouldn't throw stones." Taken literally, it means that people whose homes have walls that will shatter should not throw stones while inside. However, what this means idiomatically is that you should not be a hypocrite and should not criticize someone for something you do yourself.

Text-level comprehension is where bilingual reading strategies are key. We have mentioned elsewhere in this text about using both English-ordered signs with fingerspelled grammatical words *and* ASL translations of English print to model the connection between texts in English and meaning in ASL. Such strategies require the educational interpreter to have a high level of ASL fluency as well as additional time to model texts multiple ways.

Fingerspelling

As we know, vocabulary is a critical component of reading development. The larger your vocabulary, the larger your ability to comprehend the variety of texts that you read. In fact, vocabulary is its own independent predictor of how well you can read. The more words you know, the more easily you can read. This is one of the reasons why fingerspelling is an important aspect of literacy instruction for Deaf children.

Fingerspelling provides a link to English print (Alawad & Musyoka, 2018; Allen, 2015; Haptonstall-Nykaza & Schick, 2007; Roos, 2013; Stone, Kartheiser, Hauser, Petitto, & Allen, 2015). However, just fingerspelling a word without any other context is insufficient to support word comprehension. Fingerspelling must be connected to a concept in some way. It may be connected to a lexical sign, to a description, to depiction (classifiers), or to other words in the text. This is referred to as "chaining," or "sandwiching" (Humphries & MacDougall, 1999). You may have heard it described as sign-fingerspell-sign, or fingerspell-sign-fingerspell. The idea is that fingerspelling is presented with a signed concept of similar meaning. By embedding fingerspelling of specific English words into your interpretations, you are exposing Deaf students to more English vocabulary in context.

Strategic fingerspelling is a transitional bridge between ASL and English bilingualism (for additional specific strategies to connect ASL to printed text see Berke, 2013). Fingerspelling improves Deaf students' English literacy and new vocabulary all while helping students decode, read, and write English.

This does not mean, though, that most things should be fingerspelled. Certainly, educational interpreters should fingerspell proper nouns, technical vocabulary, abbreviations, acronyms, and use fingerspelling for emphasis or clarification. Proper nouns are particularly essential such as teachers' names, student names, etc. Educational interpreters do a disservice to Deaf students when they do not frequently fingerspell the names of the relevant parties. Using invented sign names prevents Deaf students from imprinting that person's proper name in English. Furthermore, sign names are a cultural provenance of Deaf people, so educational interpreters should not create sign names for teachers and students in the classroom.

New and/or technical vocabulary becomes *key vocabulary* the Deaf student is expected to learn and apply. When dealing with key vocabulary, fingerspelling should be didactically produced (teacher-like), slow and clear, not colloquially produced (chat-like). This means an educational interpreter must analyze the incoming message to gauge what information is critical for literacy development and/or testing in order to use fingerspelling strategically and appropriately.

See Fitzmaurice (2024) for a more thorough description of the importance of fingerspelling for educational interpreters. A caveat, though, is fingerspelling needs to be done strategically by educational interpreters and not to cover up a lack of either content knowledge or sign vocabulary (Nicodemus & Emmorey, 2015).

Sign Systems

As an educational interpreter, your responsibility is to use and model *language* with Deaf children. However, when working in educational settings, you will come across multiple visual/manual communication systems that are not actually languages. These have all arisen as attempts to teach Deaf children in a post-Milan world, particularly among educators who are not fluent in ASL. Recall that language and communication are different. Communication systems are ways of getting your point across to another without the rich capacity of language for cultural transmission, displacement, abstraction, duality, and so on. We will address some of the most common visual/manual communication systems below. Some of these are intended to be communication systems for instruction, whereas others are intended to be more like visual supplements to a spoken language. These systems are always in use to attempt to teach Deaf children English literacy without bilingual instructional methods, and thus rely to varying degrees on the phonology, morphology, and syntax of English (Moser et al., 1960).

Visual/Manual Communication Systems

One of the most common non-ASL visual/manual communication systems is Signing Exact English (SEE II), also called "Signed English" (Gustason, Pfetzing, & Zawolkow, 1980). It was developed with the intention of teaching Deaf children to read English. However, it has not been successful, largely because it has been applied to teaching Deaf children who do not have a first language foundation. SEE II is a system of signs, many of which are borrowed from ASL and then initialized, following English sentence structure. Initialization is the process of changing the handshape of a sign so that it matches the first letter of the corresponding English printed word. SEE II is intended to be a manual code for English.

In SEE II, each sign corresponds to a single English word rather than to a concept, and affixes are added to represent English morphology such as -ING and -ED. Therefore, words with the same underlying concept such as PURE, CLEAN, HOLY each have different signs, whereas in a natural signed language there is one sign for the concept of something being clean with morphological variations that indicate tense, aspect, plurality, etc. This system of affixation makes SEE II cumbersome to process from a psycholinguistic perspective, so individuals who use SEE II for long periods of time or who learn it as young children naturally adapt how they produce it so that it looks more language-like. SEE II is not culturally transmitted, and it is not productive in its own right because it is a code for English. Therefore, SEE II is not a language and nearly impossible to use effectively while interpreting (Krause & Hague, 2020; Livingston, Singer, & Abramson, 1994; Winston, 2004).

You may be wondering why SEE II is called such and not just "SEE." Often, people will refer to SEE meaning SEE II, but there is another form of SEE called

Seeing Essential English (SEE I) that was developed first and SEE II branched off of SEE I. SEE I was a system of signs for English morphemes (roots and affixes) such that each English word could be represented by a series of signs (Luetke-Stahlman & Milburn, 1996). For example, -CEPT was one sign, and the word deception was signed using DE-, -CEPT, -TION and except was signed using EX-, -CEPT, and accept with AC-, -CEPT (see Luetke-Stahlman & Milburn, 1996 for more examples). With SEE I, any English words that shared two of three characteristics (spelling, meaning, sound) were signed the same way. This creates substantial semantic confusion. For example, the word "mean" was always signed one way regardless of its use in expressions such as "words mean…" or "that person is mean…". Like SEE II, SEE I is not a language. It is a Manual Code for English (MCE).

As we mentioned in the Preface, another communication system that is quite common is the poorly named Pidgin Sign English (PSE). Again, PSE is wrongly labeled and is a Contact sign system that uses ASL signs in English grammatical order (Lucas & Valli, 1989; Monikowski, 2004). We will refer to it as Contact Sign here even though it is commonly labeled in the interpreting community as PSE. Contact Sign uses space, classifiers, and other linguistic features of ASL beyond just individual lexical signs, but the order of signs predominantly follows the order of English sentence structure, borrowed heavily from MCE, which is itself a code for English.

Though it is called "pidgin," it is not linguistically a pidgin. In linguistics, a pidgin is a contact variety of two languages that arises when there is frequent interaction between speakers of those languages. When a pidgin is passed generationally, the resulting language is called a creole (Holm, 2000; Siegel, 2008; Thomason, 2001). PSE is not linguistically considered a creole because it is not rule-governed, nor is it a native language of Deaf people, nor is it a true pidgin. However, it is a common contact variety in the Deaf community (Lucas, Bayley, & Valli, 2001). Deaf people often refer to "code switching"—the way in which they adapt their grammar to the fluency of the people they are talking to.

Another common communication system you will encounter is Conceptually Accurate Signed English (CASE). CASE is more English-like than PSE because it uses ASL signs but does not use classifiers and other complex visual structures that are part of ASL grammar. It is more language-like than SEE I or SEE II because it is not a code of English but it still relies on a knowledge of English and/or ASL to be decoded. It is extremely challenging to interpret effectively using CASE.

Simultaneous Communication (SimCom)

Simultaneous Communication (SimCom) means that information is being spoken and signed at the same time (Marschark, Lang, & Albertini, 2002). It is well documented by researchers that the spoken message and the signed message are not equivalent, and the comprehension rates of Deaf adults directly reflect the discrepancies in SimCom.

Unfortunately, SimCom is based on the notion that equivalent and/or complementary information can be communicated directly and simultaneously to both hearing and Deaf people. This is simply not the case (Cokely, 1990; Handspeak, n.d.; Tevenal & Villanueva, 2009; Whitehead, Schiavetti, MacKenzie, & Metz, 2004). Invariably, Deaf people are always missing a lot of information with SimCom as they are not getting good English to lipread, nor good ASL that makes sense.

We strongly recommend avoiding the use of SimCom whenever possible, with one exception. If the educational interpreter is speaking to someone else directly and wants to ensure the Deaf student has the gist of what the conversation is about, they can SimCom. For example, if the educational interpreter is speaking directly to the teacher while the Deaf student is present, this would be a time to use SimCom. Or, if the educational interpreter is directly advocating for a Deaf student (we will discuss this in chapter seven), those interactions should be SimCommed. If a hearing student asks the educational interpreter a question or asks about sign language, that would be a great time to SimCom. Better yet, interpret the question and provide the Deaf student an opportunity to educate their peer! Again, we realize SimCom never provides complete, meaningful access to the conversation, but if we as educational interpreters are directly interacting with hearing people in the Deaf student's presence, for those interactions we should use SimCom in an effort to include the Deaf student. It is always a good idea to reinterpret the information following the SimCom interaction as well, to ensure the Deaf student gets a clear message.

DC: I feel compelled to note that interpreters have a bad habit of using SimCom to talk to one another even when the only people present in the conversation are all hearing or all signers (such as other interpreters). For the sake of your language, PICK ONE. If you are in the habit of using SimCom in conversation, you will not be able to develop expressive fluency in ASL. SimCom should be used sparingly.

Visual Supplements to Spoken Language

One supplemental visual system that you will see is Cued Speech (also called Cueing or Cued Language) (Nicholls & Ling, 1982). Cued Speech is not a system of signs the way that PSE, SEE I, SEE II, and CASE are. Cued Speech is the use of hand signals or cues by the mouth in order to make the invisible parts of speech in English more visible. There are many speech sounds in spoken English (and other languages too) that cannot be easily distinguished by lip movements. Cued Speech supports the efforts of lipreading by providing visual cues to the Deaf person. However, not many Deaf individuals use Cued Speech as it limits access and belonging (Humphries et al., 2012; LaSasso, Crain, & Leybaert, 2003; Snoddon, 2008).

Another system that is somewhat similar to Cued Speech, but more restricted in its usage, is Visual Phonics. Visual Phonics is a system of symbols that each represent one of the phonemic sounds of the English language (Trezek & Malmgren, 2005; Smith & Wang, 2010). Visual Phonics is popular in literacy instruction with Deaf children, and some educational interpreters have learned the system of Visual Phonics to incorporate it into their interpreting during literacy instruction. However, this is a point of contention in Deaf Education, particularly among Deaf educators, and there are no empirically valid findings that it actually improves literacy for Deaf students (Cacciato, 2022; Kart, 2021; Narr, 2008; Wuestner, 2018).

SF: Some studies suggest Visual Phonics works well for some Deaf students. However, I find that the bilingual-bicultural approach (learning English through fully formed ASL) paired with extensive fingerspelling has a rich legacy of promoting literacy for Deaf children. I work with many Deaf professional colleagues with advanced degrees who learned to read effectively this way. This, however, counters the phonics-based literacy instruction we use in schools. I am also well aware that Deaf students generally have fundamental gaps in ASL and teaching them another coding system seems like time that could be better spent learning ASL.

Summary

This chapter emphasized the critical distinction between language, modality, and communication, especially in the context of Deaf education. Language is a rule-governed system essential for cognitive development, whereas modality refers to how language is expressed (e.g., spoken or signed). Communication conveys intent but doesn't necessarily involve language, such as body language. Early language exposure is crucial, as it impacts cognitive and linguistic abilities during the critical acquisition period (first five years of life). Language deprivation, common in Deaf children who lack access to a natural language, can lead to cognitive deficits, impacting their ability to comprehend abstract ideas and interact socially. Interpreters alone cannot resolve these deficits, as language acquisition requires interactive modeling.

Deaf children often experience delays in executive function and Theory of Mind, which affects social understanding. Early language acquisition, particularly of ASL, helps improve these skills, though Deaf children still face challenges such as missing incidental learning. Cochlear implants don't necessarily improve Theory of Mind outcomes.

In terms of literacy, Deaf students' reading and writing skills depend on a strong language foundation. Without it, their reading comprehension suffers, as the SVR model illustrates. Phonics-based methods are less effective for Deaf students, who rely on whole-word approaches. Educational interpreters need to assess comprehension, address vocabulary gaps, and support text-level understanding, particularly when idiomatic or figurative language is involved.

Fingerspelling plays an important role in supporting Deaf children's literacy by connecting ASL concepts to English print. Fingerspelling should be paired with signed concepts (chaining) to provide context and bridge ASL-English bilingualism. Proper nouns, technical vocabulary, and key terms should be fingerspelled clearly, but it must be done strategically to enhance literacy development rather than cover a lack of sign knowledge.

We also highlighted the shortcomings of visual/manual systems (e.g., SEE II, SimCom) that focus on English structure but lack the complexity of natural languages like ASL. These systems, often used in education, do not support true language acquisition, thus impacting cognitive and literacy development.

Thought Questions

1 What are the long-term effects of language deprivation on Deaf students, and how can educational interpreters work within their role to mitigate these effects while promoting language development and self-advocacy?
2 How does a strong foundation in ASL contribute to the literacy development of Deaf students? How could fingerspelling combined with signed concepts be used effectively to enhance a Deaf student's literacy development?
3 Compare and contrast the effectiveness of phonics-based reading instruction with whole-word approaches for Deaf students, using evidence from the chapter to support your analysis.
4 Analyze how language deprivation affects executive function and Theory of Mind development in Deaf children and explain how early ASL exposure might mitigate these effects.
5 How does the critical period for language acquisition impact Deaf children's language development? What are the implications of the critical period for educational interpreters?

References

Alawad, H., & Musyoka, M. (2018). Examining the effectiveness of fingerspelling in improving the vocabulary and literacy skills of deaf students. *Creative Education*, 9(3), 456–468.

Allen, T. E. (2015). ASL skills, fingerspelling ability, home communication context and early alphabetic knowledge of preschool-aged deaf children. *Sign Language Studies*, 15 (3), 233–265.

Allen, T. E., Letteri, A., Choi, S. H., & Dang, D. (2014). Early visual language exposure and emergent literacy in preschool deaf children: Findings from a national longitudinal study. *American Annals of the Deaf*, 159(4), 346–358.

Beck, I. L., & McKeown, M. G. (2007). Increasing young low-income children's oral vocabulary repertoires through rich and focused instruction. *The Elementary School Journal*, 107(3), 251–271. doi:10.1086/511706.

Berke, M. (2013). Reading books with young deaf children: Strategies for mediating between American Sign Language and English. *Journal of Deaf Studies and Deaf Education*, 18(3), 299–311.

Cacciato, C. (2022). Visual Phonics: An effective instructional tool for d/Deaf and hard of hearing students. *Journal of Student Scholarship*, 24, 1–6.

Caselli, N. K., Hall, W. C., & Henner, J. (2020). American Sign Language interpreters in public schools: An illusion of inclusion that perpetuates language deprivation. *Maternal and Child Health Journal*, 24(11), 1323–1329.

Cerney, B. (2007). Language acquisition, language teaching, and the interpreter as a model for language input. http://www.handandmind.org/LgAcquisition.pdf.

Cheng, Q., Roth, A., Halgren, E., & Mayberry, R. I. (2019). Effects of early language deprivation on brain connectivity: Language pathways in deaf native and late first-language learners of American Sign Language. *Frontiers in Human Neuroscience*, 13: 320.

Cokely, D. (1990). The effectiveness of three means of communication in the college classroom. *Sign Language Studies*, 69, 415–442.

Collins, A. M., & Quillian, M. R. (1969). Retrieval time from semantic memory. *Journal of Verbal Learning and Verbal Behavior*, 8(2), 240–247.

Courtin, C., Melot, A.-M., & Corroyer, D. (2008). Achieving efficient learning: Why understanding theory of mind is essential for deaf children…and their teachers. In M. Marschark & P. C. Hauser (Eds.), *Deaf cognition: Foundations and outcomes* (pp. 102–130). New York: Oxford University Press.

Ehri, L. C. (2005). Development of the ability to read words: An overview. In S. B. Neuman & D. K. Dickinson (Eds.), *Handbook of early literacy research* (Vol. 2, pp. 135–154). New York: Guilford Press.

Fitzmaurice, S. B. (2024). Importance of fingerspelling in education settings. In J. Bentley-Sassaman, R. F. Minor, & S. Fitzmaurice (Eds.), *A survey of American Sign Language/English interpreting settings* (pp. 19–32). OER Commons.

Friedmann, N., & Rusou, D. (2015). Critical period for first language: The crucial role of input during the first year of life. *Current Opinion in Neurobiology*, 35, 27–34.

Fromkin, V., Rodman, R., & Hyams, N. (2018). *An introduction to language* (11th ed.). Boston, MA: Cengage Learning.

Gough, P. B., & Tunmer, W. E. (1986). Decoding, reading, and reading disability. *Remedial and Special Education*, 7(1), 6–10.

Gulati, S. (2019). Language deprivation syndrome. In N. S. Glickman & W. C. Hall (Eds.), *Language deprivation and deaf mental health* (pp. 25–44). New York: Routledge.

Gustason, G., Pfetzing, D., & Zawolkow, E. (1980). *Signing Exact English*. Los Alamitos, CA: Modern Signs Press.

Hale, C. M., & Tager-Flusberg, H. (2003). The influence of language on theory of mind: A training study. *Developmental Science*, 6(3), 346–359.

Hall, M. L., Hall, W. C., & Caselli, N. K. (2019). Deaf children need language, not (just) speech. *First Language*, 39(4), 367–395.

Hall, W. C. (2017). What you don't know can hurt you: The risk of language deprivation by impairing sign language development in deaf children. *Maternal and Child Health Journal*, 21(5), 961–965.

Hall, W. C., Levin, L. L., & Anderson, M. L. (2017). Language deprivation syndrome: A possible neurodevelopmental disorder with sociocultural origins. *Social Psychiatry and Psychiatric Epidemiology*, 52(6), 761–776.

Handspeak. (n.d.). Simultaneous communication to use or to avoid? Handspeak. https://www.handspeak.com/learn/353/.

Haptonstall-Nykaza, T., & Schick, B. (2007). The transition from fingerspelling to English print: Facilitating English decoding. *Journal of Deaf Studies and Deaf Education*, 12(2), 172–183.

Hauser, P. C., Lukomski, J., & Hillman, T. (2008). Development of deaf and hard-of-hearing students' executive function. In M. Marschark & P. C. Hauser (Eds.), *Deaf cognition: Foundations and outcomes* (pp. 286–308). New York: Oxford University Press.

Hoff, E. (2013). *Language development* (5th ed.). Wadsworth: Cengage Learning.

Holm, J. (2000). *An introduction to pidgins and creoles*. Cambridge: Cambridge University Press.

Hoover, W. A., & Gough, P. B. (1990). The simple view of reading. *Reading and Writing*, 2(2), 127–160.

Humphries, T., Kushalnagar, P., Mathur, G., Napoli, D. J., Padden, C., Rathmann, C., & Smith, S. R. (2012). Language acquisition for deaf children: Reducing the harms of zero tolerance to the use of alternative approaches. *Harm Reduction Journal*, 13(1): 16.

Humphries, T., & MacDougall, F. (1999). Chaining and other links: Making connections between American Sign Language and English in two types of school settings. *Visual Anthropology Review*, 15(2), 84–94.

International Phonetic Association. (1999). *Handbook of the International Phonetic Association: A guide to the use of the International Phonetic Alphabet*. Cambridge: Cambridge University Press.

Johnson, R. E., Liddell, S. K., & Erting, C. J. (1989). Unlocking the curriculum: Principles for achieving access in deaf education. Gallaudet Research Institute Working Paper 89–3. Washington, DC: Gallaudet University.

Kart, A. N. (2021). Systematic review of studies on visual phonics. *Communication Disorders Quarterly*, 43(4), 261–271.

Kecskes, I. (2015). How does a learner understand idioms in a second language? In I. Kecskes (Ed.), *Intention, common ground and the egocentric speaker-hearer* (pp. 145–162). Berlin: De Gruyter Mouton.

Knoors, H., & Marschark, M. (2014). *Teaching deaf learners: Psychological and developmental foundations*. New York: Oxford University Press.

Krause, J. C., & Hague, A. K. (2020). Signing Exact English transliteration: Effects of accuracy and lag time on message intelligibility. *Journal of Deaf Studies and Deaf Education*, 25(2), 199–211.

Langer, E. C., & Schick, B. (2004, October). How accessible is classroom discourse to deaf children using educational interpreters? Paper presented at the Colorado Symposium on Deafness, Language, and Learning, Colorado Springs, CO.

LaSasso, C., Crain, K., & Leybaert, J. (2003). Rhyme generation in deaf students: The effect of exposure to cued speech. *Journal of Deaf Studies and Deaf Education*, 8(3), 250–270.

LEAD-K. (n.d.). Language Equality and Acquisition for Deaf Kids. Retrieved April 28, 2025, from https://www.lead-k.org.

Lenneberg, E. H. (1967). *Biological foundations of language*. New York: Wiley.

Livingston, S., Singer, B., & Abramson, T. (1994). Effectiveness compared: ASL interpretation vs. transliteration. *Sign Language Studies*, 82, 1–54.

Lucas, C., Bayley, R., & Valli, C. (2001). *Sociolinguistic variation in American Sign Language*. Washington, DC: Gallaudet University Press.

Lucas, C., & Valli, C. (1989). Language contact in the American deaf community. In C. Lucas (Ed.), *The sociolinguistics of the Deaf community* (pp. 11–40). Cambridge, MA: Academic Press.

Luetke-Stahlman, B., & Milburn, W. O. (1996). A history of Seeing Essential English (SEE I). *American Annals of the Deaf*, 141(1), 29–34.

Marschark, M., & Hauser, P. C. (2008). The impact of language experience on the development of theory of mind in deaf children. In M. Marschark & P. Hauser (Eds.), *Deaf cognition: Foundations and outcomes* (pp. 139–155). New York: Oxford University Press.

Marschark, M., & Hauser, P. C. (2012). *How deaf children learn: What parents and teachers need to know*. New York: Oxford University Press.

Marschark, M., & Knoors, H. (2012). Educating deaf children: Language, cognition, and learning. *Deafness & Education International*, 14(3), 136–160.

Marschark, M., Lang, H. G., & Albertini, J. A. (2002). *Educating deaf students: From research to practice*. New York: Oxford University Press.

Marschark, M., Sapere, P., Convertino, C., & Seewagen, R. (2005). Educational interpreting: Access and outcomes. In M. Marschark, R. Peterson, & E. Winston (Eds.), *Sign language interpreting and interpreter education* (pp. 57–83). New York: Oxford University Press.

Marschark, M., & Spencer, P. E. (2009). *Evidence of best practice models and outcomes in the education of deaf and hard-of-hearing children: An international review*. Trim: National Council for Special Education.

Marschark, M., & Wauters, L. (2008). Language comprehension and learning by deaf students. In M. Marschark & P. C. Hauser (Eds.), *Deaf cognition: Foundations and outcomes* (pp. 309–350). New York: Oxford University Press.

Mayberry, R. I. (2002). Cognitive development in deaf children: The interface of language and perception in neuropsychology. *Handbook of Neuropsychology*, 8, 71–107.

Mayberry, R. I. (2007). When timing is everything: Age of first-language acquisition effects on second-language learning. *Applied Psycholinguistics*, 28(3), 537–549. doi:10.1017/S0142716407070294.

Mayberry, R. I., del Giudice, A. A., & Lieberman, A. M. (2011). Reading achievement in relation to phonological coding and awareness in deaf readers: A meta-analysis. *Journal of Deaf Studies and Deaf Education*, 16(2), 164–188.

Mayberry, R. I., & Locke, E. (2003). Age constraints on first versus second language acquisition: Evidence for linguistic plasticity and epigenesis. *Brain and Language*, 87(3), 369–384.

McCardle, P., Scarborough, H. S., & Catts, H. W. (2001). Predicting, explaining, and preventing children's reading difficulties. *Learning Disabilities Research & Practice*, 16(4), 230–239.

McQuarrie, L., & Abbott, M. (2013). Bilingual deaf students' phonological awareness in ASL and reading skills in English. *Sign Language Studies*, 14(1), 80–100.

Meier, R. P. (2002). The acquisition of verb agreement: Pointing out arguments for the linguistic status of agreement in sign languages. In G. Morgan & B. Woll (Eds.), *Directions in sign language acquisition* (pp. 115–141). Amsterdam: John Benjamins.

Monikowski, C. (2004). Language myths in interpreted education: First language, second language, what language? In E. A. Winston (Ed.), *Educational interpreting: How it can succeed* (pp. 48–60). Washington, DC: Gallaudet University Press.

Morford, J. P., & Carlson, M. L. (2011). Sign perception and recognition in non-native signers of ASL. *Language Learning and Development*, 7(2), 149–168.

Morford, J. P., & Mayberry, R. I. (2000). A reexamination of "early exposure" and its implications for language acquisition by eye. In C. Chamberlain, J. P. Morford, & R. I. Mayberry (Eds.), *Language acquisition by eye* (pp. 111–127). Mahwah, NJ: Erlbaum.

Moser, H. M., O'Neill, J. J., Oyer, H. J., Wolfe, S. M., Abernathy, E. A., & Schowe Jr, B. M. (1960). Historical aspects of manual communication. *Journal of Speech and Hearing Disorders*, 25(2), 145–151.

Mounty, J. L., Pucci, C. T., & Harmon, K. C. (2013). How deaf American Sign Language/English bilingual children become proficient readers: An emic perspective. *Journal of Deaf Studies and Deaf Education*, 19(3), 333–346.

Narr, R. F. (2008). Phonological awareness and decoding in deaf/hard-of-hearing students who use Visual Phonics. *Journal of Deaf Studies and Deaf Education*, 13(3), 405–416.

National Association of the Deaf. (n.d.). Implications of language deprivation for young deaf, DeafBlind, DeafDisabled, and hard of hearing children. Silver Spring, MD: National Association of the Deaf. https://www.nad.org/implications-of-language-deprivation-for-young-deaf-deafblind-deafdisabled-and-hard-of-hearing-children.

National Institute of Child Health and Human Development. (2000). *Report of the National Reading Panel: Teaching children to read: An evidence-based assessment of the scientific research literature on reading and its implications for reading instruction* (NIH Publication No. 00–4769). Washington, DC: U.S. Government Printing Office.

Nicholls, G. H., & Ling, D. (1982). Cued speech and the reception of spoken language. *Journal of Speech and Hearing Research*, 25(2), 262–269.

Nicodemus, B., & Emmorey, K. (2015). Directionality in ASL-English interpreting: Accuracy and articulation quality in L1 and L2. *Interpreting*, 17(2), 145–166.

Owens, R. E. (2016). *Language development: An introduction* (9th ed.). London: Pearson.

Peterson, C. C., & Slaughter, V. P. (2006). Telling the story of theory of mind: Deaf and hearing children's narratives and mental state understanding. *British Journal of Developmental Psychology*, 24(1), 151–179.

Peterson, R., & Monikowski, C. (2010). Perceptions of efficacy of sign language interpreters working in K–12 settings. In K. M. Christensen (Ed.), *Ethical considerations in educating children who are deaf or hard of hearing* (pp. 129–153). Washington, DC: Gallaudet University Press.

Petitto, L. A., Katerelos, M., Levy, B., Gauna, K., Tetrault, K., & Ferraro, V. (2001). Bilingual signed and spoken language acquisition from birth: Implications for the mechanisms underlying early bilingual language acquisition. *Journal of Child Language*, 28(2), 453–496.

Roos, C. (2013). Young deaf children's fingerspelling in learning to read and write: An ethnographic study in a signing setting. *Deafness & Education International*, 15(3), 149–178.

Schick, B. (2004). How might learning through an educational interpreter influence cognitive development? In E. A. Winston (Ed.), *Educational interpreting: How it can succeed* (pp. 73–87). Washington, DC: Gallaudet University Press.

Schick, B. (2008). A model of learning within an interpreted K–12 educational setting. In M. Marschark & P. Hauser (Eds.), *Deaf cognition: Foundations and outcomes* (pp. 351–386). New York: Oxford University Press.

Schick, B., de Villiers, P., de Villiers, J., & Hoffmeister, R. (2007). Language and theory of mind: A study of deaf children. *Child Development*, 78(2), 376–396.

Siegel, J. (2008). *The emergence of pidgin and creole languages*. Oxford: Oxford University Press.

Smith, A., & Wang, Y. (2010). The impact of Visual Phonics on the phonological awareness and speech production of a student who is deaf: A case study. *American Annals of the Deaf*, 155(2), 124–130.

Snoddon, K. (2008). American Sign Language and early intervention. *Canadian Modern Language Review*, 64(4), 581–604.

Snoddon, K., Small, A., & Cripps, J. (2004). *A parent guidebook: ASL and early literacy*. Mississauga, Ontario: Ampersand Printing.

Snow, C. E. (2002). *Reading for understanding: Toward an R&D program in reading comprehension*. Santa Monica, CA: RAND Corporation.

Stone, A., Kartheiser, G., Hauser, P., Petitto, L., & Allen, T. (2015). Fingerspelling as a novel gateway into reading fluency in deaf bilinguals. *PLoS ONE*, 10(10): e0139610.

Tevenal, S., & Villanueva, M. (2009). Are you getting the message? The effects of SimCom on the message received by deaf, hard of hearing, and hearing students. *Sign Language Studies*, 9(3), 266–286.

Thomason, S. G. (2001). *Language contact: An introduction*. Washington, DC: Georgetown University Press.

Trezek, B. J., & Malmgren, K. W. (2005). The efficacy of utilizing a phonics treatment package with middle school deaf and hard-of-hearing students. *Journal of Deaf Studies and Deaf Education*, 10(3), 256–271.

Valli, C., Lucas, C., Mulrooney, K. J., & Villanueva, M. (2011). *Linguistics of American Sign Language: An introduction* (5th ed.). Washington, DC: Gallaudet University Press.

Wellman, H. M., & Liu, D. (2004). Scaling of theory-of-mind tasks. *Child Development*, 75(2), 523–541.

Whitehead, R. L., Schiavetti, N., MacKenzie, D. J., & Metz, D. E. (2004). Intelligibility of speech produced during simultaneous communication. *Journal of Communication Disorders*, 37(3), 241–253.

Winston, E. A. (2004). Interpretability and accessibility of mainstream classrooms. In E. A. Winston (Ed.), *Educational interpreting: How it can succeed* (pp. 15–36). Washington, DC: Gallaudet University Press.

Wuestner, M. (2018). Critical review: Does a literacy program with Visual Phonics improve phonological awareness and phonics skills in d/Deaf or hard of hearing children aged 3-9? [Unpublished manuscript]. University of Western Ontario. https://www.uwo.ca/fhs/lwm/teaching/EBP/2018_19/Wuestner.pdf.

Yule, G. (2020). *The study of language* (8th ed.). Cambridge: Cambridge University Press.

7 Interpreting Processes and Decision-Making

Community and educational interpreters differ primarily in purpose, audience, and role. Community interpreters typically work with adults in settings focusing on equal access through neutral message delivery. In contrast, educational interpreters work with Deaf students—often still developing language skills—in school settings where they support both communication and learning. Their role extends beyond interpreting to include advocacy, collaboration with the Individualized Education Program (IEP) Team, and instructional support, requiring a more adaptive and student-centered approach.

This chapter delves into the evolving interpreter metaphors that have guided the professional understanding of the role of educational interpreters and illustrating the complexities and cognitive demands inherent in their work. Traditionally viewed through the lens of metaphors like the *Helper* or *Conduit* metaphors, these representations have often oversimplified the interpreter's responsibilities, leading to misunderstandings of their role in educational settings. As these metaphors have evolved, new models such as the *Facilitator* and *Bilingual-Bicultural* metaphors have emerged, each attempting to address the diverse and active contributions interpreters make. However, none of these models have fully captured the dynamic nature of the work. This chapter examines the *Partners in Education (PIE) Role Metaphor* as a more comprehensive framework, recognizing the interpreter's multifaceted contributions as educators, communicators, advocates, and team members within the school environment.

The chapter also examines key interpreting models—such as *Skopos Theory, Gile's Effort Model, Cokely's Sociolinguistic Model*, and *Russell's Meaning-Based Model*—to inform decision-making that considers both cognitive demands and contextual requirements. Additionally, the *Gish Model, Demand-Control Schema (DCS)*, and *Role Space Framework* are emphasized for their practical use in educational settings, helping interpreters make ethical, student-focused decisions.

Finally, the chapter explores ethical considerations by comparing the National Association of the Deaf and Registry of Interpreters for the Deaf (NAD-RID) Code of Professional Conduct (CPC) with the Educational Interpreter Code of Ethics (EICOE). It highlights the importance of ethical adaptability, cultural humility, and thoughtful reflection when addressing value

DOI: 10.4324/9781003423058-7

conflicts, autonomy, and collaboration within the IEP Team. Ultimately, the chapter advocates for evidence-based, context-sensitive frameworks that recognize the complex and vital role of educational interpreters and the necessity to adapt and employ a student-centered approach in their role.

Interpreter Metaphors and Roles

Although interpreting is a fairly young profession, we have seen many metaphors used to describe the act of interpreting. Many metaphors have fallen out of favor because they struggle to capture what our work should look like and are often in direct opposition to the preceding metaphors' application.

Many texts refer to these metaphors as interpreting models. Certainly, all metaphors are models in some way; however, models tend to provide relative descriptions of interpreting and/or interpretation processes. Think of a model airplane as a scaled-down version of a real airplane. A model would reflect what interpreters actually do, a daunting task because so much of the interpreter's work is cognitive. Metaphors, however, generally compare and label an interpreter's actions with something we already know. Metaphors tend to be very simplified ways to describe how we function in our work without actually describing the interpreting process itself.

Helper Metaphor

Shortly after the launch of the Registry of Interpreters for the Deaf (RID)—which you will likely have learned about in other courses—the ASL-English interpreting field took hold. Most interpreters at that time were volunteers and more than willing to help Deaf people access the world around them. From that notion, the *Helper Metaphor* was born. This metaphor focused on the interpreter's role and situated interpreters as becoming overly involved with Deaf adults by providing advice, direction, or even teaching. The underpinning of this role metaphor was an assumption Deaf people could not take care of their own business and was, frankly, paternalistic.

The *Helper Metaphor* for interpreters is rarely seen any more in the professional interpreting community except among the educational interpreter community. Naturally, as educational interpreters, we tend to feel we want to be helpful by becoming friends with the Deaf student, helping them with homework, and generally taking care of the Deaf student's needs. With younger children, of course, they need more general help, but the caveat is to wean Deaf students from dependency on external support toward autonomy in which they can function in a self-sufficient manner. We have both witnessed educational interpreters unable to reduce the amount of helpfulness or mothering, and graduating Deaf teens who are ill-equipped to deal with the world outside of the school classroom. A significant contributing factor is educational interpreters who continue to enact a *Helper Metaphor*, which ultimately sets up the Deaf person to fail in life.

Conduit Metaphor

To directly counter the *Helper Metaphor*, community interpreters shifted to the *Conduit Metaphor*. Sometimes it is also referred to as a "machine metaphor" in that interpreters were expected to be a machine-like service—detached, neutral, objective, and impersonal (Lee, Winston, & Forestal, 2023). Educational interpreters were merely conduits of information—much like a telephone. We all know verbatim transmission is impossible, yet that was what was and is expected.

Unfortunately, we know interpreters cannot be translation machines and could not meet that expectation. In fact, our very presence changes the dynamic of the communication event. Nevertheless, we still see interpreters trying to enact this type of metaphor. We can observe this metaphor in a number of ways, not only in terms of how interpreters do their jobs, but also in the way that they talk about their work. For instance, interpreters sometimes use phrases such as, "I'm just going to interpret exactly what you say," "My goal is to be invisible" (which makes us laugh as individuals who use a visual language), or the seemingly benign "I'm just the interpreter." These expressions all feed into the notion we are translation conduit-machines, not participants in the communication event, and instead serve solely as a means by which information moves unaltered between two parties.

Another major challenge to the *Conduit Metaphor* is evident in phrases such as, "My job is to convey your meaning." This overlooks a key premise that educational interpreters do not transmit fixed meanings but instead infer and reconstruct intended meanings based on the signs, speech, or behavior of others. Meaning is neither tangible nor directly observable; it is inherently unstable and context-dependent. Rather than being transferred intact, meanings are co-constructed through interaction, with interpreters relying on contextual cues to make the most relevant inferences possible.

Our goal as educational interpreters is to preserve intended meaning—not the original form—by interpreting expressions as cognitive prompts that guide us toward a speaker's intent. It may sound complex—and it is—because interpreting is not about decoding words, but about inferring meaning within a shared cognitive and communicative space.

Suffice to say, educational interpreters also do not work in a machine-like manner by decoding, transferring, and re-encoding classroom communication. As educational interpreters, we are active humans in the classrooms where we work. One reason educational interpreters need to be careful about how they characterize their work is the potential impact that these ideas will have on people who rely on these services. For instance, administrators and teachers may make assumptions about the work we do and how we do it, which can have an overall negative impact. In many cases, teachers loathe educational interpreters who enact the *Conduit Metaphor* as the interpreter behaves as a machine-like instrument and not an engaged member of the classroom (Antia & Kreimeyer, 2001; Fitzmaurice, 2021).

Facilitator Metaphor

Interpreters recognized that functioning like machines was unrealistic, and many Deaf individuals also rejected the *Conduit Metaphor* for its lack of humanity and relational depth. Eventually, the *Communication Facilitator Metaphor* emerged in practice (Roy, 1993). This metaphor acknowledged the interpreter's active role in managing the physical and visual aspects of communication—such as indicating speakers, adjusting placement, improving lighting, and minimizing visual distractions—to enhance accessibility and understanding (Metzger, 1995; Roy, 2000).

At its root, though, the *Facilitator Metaphor* is still just a tweak on the *Conduit Metaphor* in that interpreters' function as a channel (albeit a communicatively clearer channel) that transfers messages from sender to receiver and back again. The *Facilitator Metaphor* failed to account for the things that interpreters did to navigate the power and social dynamics in an interpreting setting. As with the *Conduit Metaphor*, the efficacy of an interpretation was in terms of its one-to-one or word-to-sign correspondence.

Though the *Facilitator Metaphor* is generally out of favor, and its successor role metaphor, the *Bilingual-Bicultural Metaphor*, is more popular, interpreters still see the word *facilitator* as being very popular in the education system (Fitzmaurice, 2021). For example, teachers use the phrase *facilitator* to mean an educational interpreter who is flexible and fully engaged in the classroom and not functioning as a *conduit metaphor* robot—i.e. does not say "that is not my job" when asked to perform routine classroom tasks. Teachers of the Deaf in particular like the *facilitator* idea in that such educational interpreters will share information about the student and student performance with the teacher of the Deaf. This seems to be a twist on the traditional community-interpreter role metaphor, but again, it is used often by those who do not enact an educational interpreter role metaphor (see later in this chapter).

SF: I find the word facilitator to be a fair-weather friend, meaning we tend to throw it around, but it truly has an ambiguous meaning. A quick Google search yields the definition of a facilitator: "a person or thing that makes an action or process easy or easier." To be fair, as interpreters we do not make communication easier, we make it accessible or possible. We are not actually making anything happen—the hearing and Deaf participants are making the discourse happen. To pretend we are making it happen (facilitating the discourse) disempowers those parties; we are merely making their discourse accessible to each other.

Bilingual-Bicultural Metaphor

The 1990s made way for a new role metaphor, the *Bilingual-Bicultural Metaphor*, which went hand-in-hand with the push for ASL and English to be taught to Deaf children using a bilingual-bicultural method. This metaphor also paired well with research at the time acknowledging that the presence of interpreters in and of itself influences the discourse. We are neither machines nor invisible, but participants in the discourse (Roy, 2000).

Interpreters enacting the *Bilingual-Bicultural Metaphor* acknowledge power and social structures and recognize that language and culture cannot be cleanly separated (Cokely, 1992). Interpreters enacting this metaphor are acutely aware that we need to be mindful of the speaker's goal, and mediate both cultures (Deaf and hearing) and languages (ASL and English). It is of interest as noted later in this chapter that the *Gish Construct for Interpreting: A Goal-to-Detail Model of Information Processing* (*Gish Model*) was readily adopted at this time (Gish, 1987).

Although educational interpreters are aware of the social dynamics within school settings, much of the *Bilingual-Bicultural Metaphor* does not align well with their day-to-day realities. Although educational interpreters can help make resources about Deaf culture more accessible to Deaf students (see chapter five), and though many may hold other multicultural identities, most Deaf students are not bicultural in the traditional sense of navigating both Deaf and hearing cultures. Likewise, most Deaf students are not functionally bilingual in ASL and English (see chapter six).

Certainly, there are other role metaphors for interpreters. For example, the *Ally Metaphor* (Baker-Shenk, 1991), the *Advocate Metaphor* (Roy, 1993), and *the Institutional Agent Metaphor* (Davidson, 2000). However, let's turn our attention back to the educational environment.

Davino Inverted Triangles of Responsibility

None of these role metaphors work well for educational interpreters. They are all geared toward interpreters working with Deaf adults in the community. The educational interpreting field has long known the community lens, role, and actual work are vastly different and, in real terms, educational interpreters work every minute juggling a multitude of factors.

One popular, but theoretical model includes the Davino (1985) *Inverted Triangles of Responsibility* model (see Figure 7.1). This model has become de facto practice and been replicated and modified and re-replicated for the last 40 years (for example, Lawson & Hamrick, 2011). Davino put forth the idea that it is important for educational interpreters to understand a Deaf student's shifting levels of independence and responsibility. Defining responsibility or independence is troublesome. Davino did not put forth any benchmark for what constitutes independence or responsibility. As such, they are left to the construct of any educator and interpreter, potentially leading to the withdrawal of support too early or even too late.

Indeed, high school students should be more responsible or independent than elementary school students—but responsible and independent in what ways? What are responsibilities? How much independence do you need to begin adulting? And is there really a seamless transition up or down the triangle?

Nor does this model clearly represent what actually happens in a classroom. It does not address the nuanced environmental, linguistic, or systemic barriers encountered by Deaf students, nor does it address the fluidity of the educational interpreter's role.

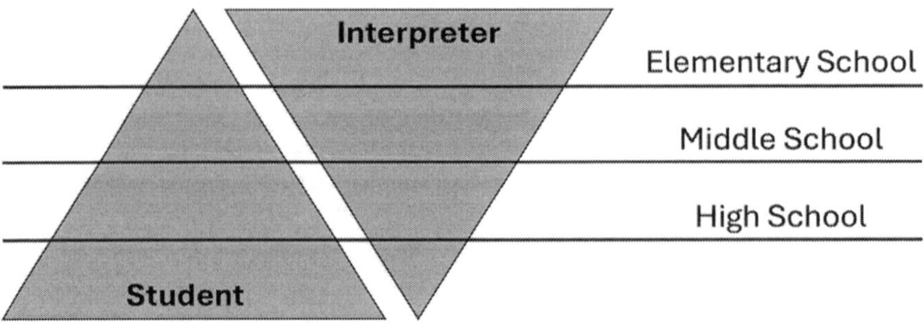

Figure 7.1 Davino Inverted Triangles of Responsibility

In addition, this model is only theoretical and has no empirical evidence to support it. Although it remains very popular, we would discourage educational interpreters from advocating this model's use.

Indeed, the specific "responsibilities" for Deaf students and educational interpreters should change as students mature, but it is not as simple as this model claims.

Partners in Education Role Metaphor

As you can see, sadly, much of the information of the educational interpreter's role was created in a vacuum without really assessing what an interpreted education entails. Often, the role was described by policy makers trying to wrongly apply the community lens into standards or guidelines for educational interpreters.

SF: To sell the idea that community-based interpreting and educational interpreting are very different, I often use the analogy that if you have heart problems you should see a cardiologist, not a neurologist. Asking a neurologist to treat your heart would generally not be a great decision. Applying cardiology practices to neurology is somewhat laughable, and most people understand that while both are sophisticated physicians, they do different work. Doctors are doctors but not all doctors have the same expertise. Educational interpreters are experts at interpreting for children and youth, which is vastly different from interpreting for adults. Interpreting is interpreting, but not all interpreters have the same expertise. It is unclear why some people struggle to recognize that difference and apply community-based (adult) interpreting standards, expectations, practices, roles, et cetera to someone who interprets in an education setting (children and youth).

There are a plethora of research articles and books examining what educational interpreters do in the classroom. Similarly, there is a lot of research on policy and guidelines for educational interpreters, the experiences of Deaf students with educational interpreters, content comprehension of Deaf students, the accessibility of classroom content and discourse, miscue analysis and content exclusion of educational interpreters, and even the efficacy of different Educational Interpreter Performance Assessment (EIPA) levels of educational interpreters.

However, educational interpreters for the most part operate moment-to-moment on their own with no clear understanding of their role and without a role metaphor appropriate for framing and explaining their work. Without a doubt, the primary responsibility for educational interpreters is always to interpret. But what about the other stuff?

The *Partners in Education (PIE) Role Metaphor* (see Figure 7.2) was designed to generally look similar to a stage. Just as a stage actor moves to different points on the stage, educational interpreters will move to enact different aspects of their role. The next sections will review each of these roles in detail.

Interpreting

You will notice first and foremost the center stage placement goes to the *Interpreting* function. This may seem like a no-brainer as that is our primary role and we have to remember interpreting supersedes all the other roles we may enact.

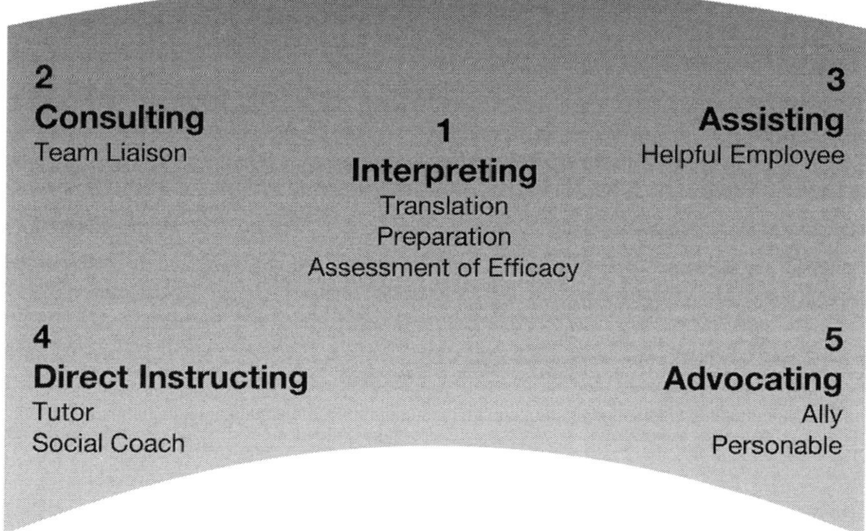

Figure 7.2 Partners in Education (PIE) Role Metaphor

Interpreting encompasses not only actual interpreting of classroom communication but also monitoring the communication between hearing peers (Tiselius & Englund Dimitrova, 2023). Sometimes we need to include the communication between peers in our interpretation and sometimes we do not. Either way, we need to be actively monitoring peer conversations. The role of interpreting in educational contexts is more expansive than the specific act of interpreting between two languages. For instance, interpreting may also include directing a student's attention to visual information in the classroom or textbook and even holding an interpretation to allow the Deaf student to look at such materials (Smith, 2013). It sometimes involves presenting some information in simpler terms.

Also, part of the *Interpreting* role is translation work, in that if a Deaf student is signing some information, we may be tasked in the student's IEP to translate that into written English. It may also include—again based on the student's IEP—translating print material such as a textbook section or worksheet into ASL.

One of the most time-consuming components of the *Interpreting* function is preparation. *Interpreting* includes preparing materials ahead of time for interpreting. Preparation includes, for example, studying a textbook chapter or short story, or looking at teacher notes. Preparation of materials takes a lot of time and goes beyond just pre-reading the materials to breaking them down (Gish, 1987) so the most salient portions are included in the interpretation. Preparation strategies are addressed in the next chapter.

Preparation also includes preparing the environment to allow the best visual access we can provide for a Deaf student. Examples of these duties include moving desks, getting things set up, making sure all the technology is working, and meeting educational team members to craft creative solutions to make the environment more accessible. If we are working with students who use technical equipment (see chapter five), we are also preparing that equipment for use with tasks such as replacing batteries, doing a listening check, and other minor troubleshooting activities.

Lastly under the *Interpreting* role, educational interpreters are also always assessing the efficacy of the interpreting. This means we are always watching the Deaf student to ensure they truly are tracking with the information. Because Deaf students often do not have language skills commensurate with their peers, we need to continually assess the students' comprehension to determine if we need to modify our interpretation or move to a different place on the role metaphor stage.

Consulting

The next position on the *PIE Role Metaphor* stage is the role of *Consulting*. If you recall from earlier in this chapter, when teachers of the Deaf use the word "*facilitator*" they refer to this role. Essentially, performing the *Consulting* role means keeping members of the educational team informed about the Deaf student's progress. This role also entails letting the education team know what materials (if any) the Deaf student is struggling with, any interpreting revisions that need to be made, and any other information that may be beneficial for inclusion on the IEP. By virtue of our bilingual position and direct work with the Deaf student, we have a comprehensive lens on how the Deaf student is functioning in the mainstream environment.

Educational interpreters are generally not trained in formal student assessment practices, such as evaluating academic progress, cognitive development, or instructional effectiveness. Their expertise lies in interpreting, not in measuring learning outcomes or diagnosing educational needs. Because of this, it is imperative that educational interpreters regularly share observations with the educational team—such as whether the student appears to understand content, participates meaningfully in class discussions, or responds appropriately to assignments and instructions. These insights can be invaluable for teachers, special educators, and IEP Team members, who rely on a full picture of the student's engagement and comprehension. By collaborating closely and providing context-specific feedback, interpreters help ensure that assessment and instructional decisions are based on accurate, well-rounded information, ultimately supporting the student's academic and language development.

The *Consulting* role also includes doing some consulting duties such as guiding teachers on how to work with an educational interpreter and Deaf student and even how to make classroom activities more visually accessible for students. Often at the beginning of the year or semester, educational interpreters also provide some consulting on how a cochlear implant works, or explaining aspects of deafness, etc. Educational interpreters should refer teachers to appropriate team members (audiologist, teacher of the Deaf, etc.) and to resources from national organizations for further information (National Association of the Deaf, National Association of Interpreters in Education, etc.). As Deaf students become more independent and able to advocate for their own needs, this responsibility should shift to them. In reality, the educational interpreter should not be solely responsible for any of this information, as it should come from families, teachers of the Deaf, audiologists, and other team members. However, educational interpreters are often the easiest go-to for information. Therefore, educational interpreters should be prepared to explain some basics and ready to refer more complicated questions to the appropriate team members.

SF: For example, educational interpreters can discuss with teachers the possibility of the teacher using the whiteboard. This avoids the educational interpreter having to run to the whiteboard every time a teacher reads out a math problem. Having a teacher write out a math problem on a whiteboard creates a more authentic accommodation for all students. Even during popcorn reading (turn taking) in the classroom, educational interpreters can discuss using a soft cotton ball (one that is large enough and colorful enough to be seen) to be tossed around giving the set expectation that the person with the ball holds the floor to talk or is reading. These types of accommodations aid the Deaf student with visual clues that turn taking is occurring and promote an understanding that active participation is occurring and encouraged.

Assisting

Educational interpreters work in a larger system that reaches beyond the classroom to the school and, ultimately, the entire school district. One of the hallmarks for anyone working in the education system is the general notion of being a helpful contributor to the system—oftentimes beyond the primary scope of duties. Being a helpful employee applies to educational interpreters as well but is *never* at the expense of providing services for Deaf students. Educational interpreters are active members of a classroom and, as such, when we are not interpreting or working with the Deaf student, we can provide some general assistance to teachers or hearing students. Being helpful can include helping to prepare classroom materials, copying, or helping hearing students with their desk work. Educational interpreters, as part of a school community, may also be asked to attend to bus duty before school begins or briefly monitor the classroom if a teacher needs to step out for a moment. While this may be controversial, again, being a helpful employee is *never* at the expense of providing services for Deaf students.

SF: While working in an elementary school, to be a helpful employee, I often volunteered to do morning bus duty. As the students disembarked the school busses, I greeted each student with a big, "Good morning. Today's sign is ...." And would then select any random sign. When the Deaf student arrived, they helped me do this and ultimately, I would interpret the Deaf student taking over the showing the sign of the day (while I interpreted). This did three things. It allowed me to be a helpful employee. It also encouraged hearing students to begin signing. Lastly, it allowed an early opportunity for the Deaf student to begin sharing their language. It was also rewarding to see hearing children practicing their sign language with the Deaf students at recess. Being a helpful employee in this way always felt like a triple win.

Direct Instructing

Direct Instructing, often referred to as tutoring, is the next space on the role stage. Although educational interpreters do not hold teacher qualifications, *Direct Instructing* encompasses pre-teaching vocabulary for an upcoming lesson, teaching concepts a Deaf student may not know, and reteaching or reviewing classroom content.

Often in mainstream classes, a Deaf student may not understand the interpretation or the content material and may need some important information backfilled or to be prompted by the educational interpreter to recall what they already know. This would be deemed *Direct Instruction*. Any time an educational interpreter stops interpreting and dialogs with the student (again without interpreting), it would be considered *Direct Instructing*.

SF: Too often Deaf students are placed in mainstream classrooms without the appropriate language skills or background knowledge. What is interesting is that many educational interpreters engage in direct instruction very frequently. I have seen educational interpreters spend more time providing direct instruction than actually interpreting. It is not a bad thing per se—without direct instruction, the Deaf student would be lost. If an educational interpreter is no longer interpreting but spending time with direct instruction, this constitutes a modification of the curriculum—no longer interpreting the curriculum content in favor of direct instruction. Any modification or time spent in direct instruction should be indicated in the student's IEP and shared with the rest of the team. Unfortunately, many educational interpreters do not share that they stopped interpreting and stayed in a direct instruction role.

DC: In my experience, interpreters are actually shy of admitting that they engage in this direct instruction, because they have been trained with adult, community-oriented models of interpreting and do not think they are "supposed to" do direct instruction. The critical piece in Stephen's advice is sharing with the IEP Team. Too often, Deaf students continue in inappropriate placements because educational interpreters' work is actually masking disparities in Deaf student performance. Ultimately, the team may decide to have the educational interpreter fulfill this function, but it absolutely must be documented as modification in the IEP.

On the educational interpreter's role stage, *Direct Instructing* most often takes the form of pre-teaching or scaffolding. *Scaffolding* is when you take what the student knows and build on it to teach new concepts. Curriculum is scaffolded, but the foundation that the curriculum is built upon assumes some base level of language and knowledge about the world. The further along a student is in their education, the more language and knowledge they are expected to have. If the scaffolded curriculum does not have a foundation on which to build, it fails to support a student's learning. Deaf students are often missing language and/or knowledge, largely due to early language deprivation and/or lack of access to incidental learning. Therefore, educational interpreters find themselves filling in gaps in Deaf student language and world knowledge as a natural part of the educational interpreting process. When these gaps can be filled with brief explanations, a quick reference to an image or to a past shared experience, then the interpreter can provide scaffolds during the interpreted event (i.e., the interpreter switches seamlessly between *Direct Instructing* and *Interpreting*). A good time to do this type of scaffolding is when the teacher asks questions of the class to prompt brainstorming about what the students know before the teacher introduces a topic. This is a good time for the educational interpreter to check in with the Deaf student and to potentially add a few extra scaffolds. Educational interpreters can also use the term "scaffolding" with the teacher rather than words like "expansion" or "explanation" so that you are both on the same page about what you are doing. When Deaf student knowledge or language gaps require more intensive support, additional *Direct Instructing* must happen outside of interpreting time. At this point, educational interpreters should be documenting the concepts that need to be reviewed and working with the educational team to ensure there is time for that review.

DC: I was interpreting for a Deaf student who used spoken English as their primary receptive and expressive language. They thought Renaissance meant "reverse." That is how they interpreted the sound of the word "rebirth," which makes sense because "rebirth" is an unfamiliar term for middle school students. I was able to repair that understanding with a quick scaffold. Even when a student primarily attends to the spoken English, they will need such supports to clarify concepts they miss or misunderstand. It is important to check in with students periodically to catch and clarify these misunderstandings.

Another part of the *Direct Instructing* role is serving as a social coach by encouraging a Deaf student to answer a teacher's question, or to engage in a conversation with a peer. As a social coach, we actively support student language attempts, encourage appropriate peer interactions, address inappropriate behaviors, and praise appropriate behavior. Social coaching also means we are always seeking clues from the Deaf student to determine their ability to interact independently.

Again, nearly all educational interpreters spend time in the *Direct Instructing* role; however, often this role is hidden—particularly if an educational interpreter enacts a *Conduit Metaphor*. What is important to also acknowledge is that *Direct Instruction* depends on teaching strategies and scaffolding to backfill gaps in a Deaf student's knowledge. Educational interpreters need to share what they are doing with the team. If we withhold that information, the team makes assumptions about what the Deaf student can and cannot do. This will affect placement decisions and may result in Deaf students persisting in an inappropriate placement where they cannot receive a Free and Appropriate Public Education (FAPE).

Advocating

The last point on the role stage for educational interpreters includes working as an *Advocate* both on behalf of, and alongside, Deaf students. Younger Deaf students will not know how to advocate for themselves, so when moving into the *Advocating* role, educational interpreters need to do that in front of the Deaf student. Doing so allows younger Deaf students to witness firsthand the dynamics of advocacy and helps them form some self-advocacy skills. As Deaf students mature, educational interpreters should constantly be inviting Deaf students to lead their own self-advocacy.

Advocating can include negotiating the environment for accommodation, making interpreting requests, requests to teachers for captioned videos, and even sharing information about how to work with Deaf students. We may even consider guiding Deaf students on how to maintain their own technology and promoting their efforts at independence within this realm. Of course, once Deaf students are able to self-advocate, educational interpreters transition to being an *ally* as we support Deaf students' self-advocacy efforts.

One of the most significant extensions of this role is simply being friendly and personable with the Deaf student. Being friendly does not mean we become the Deaf students' friend, but we are human beings. Undoubtedly, educational interpreters are often the only people with whom Deaf students can easily communicate. They will want to share all that is happening in their world and educational interpreters should capitalize on this opportunity to model dialogues and encourage expressive language use. Educational interpreters who are not personable do not fit well into the education system.

SF: The flip side is also true as I have seen several educational interpreters being too personable in that they forget interpreting is paramount to our role. Such interpreters can be seen spending extensive amounts of time just chatting with the Deaf student instead of interpreting. And truth be told, some Deaf students like this, but we need to be wary of spending too much time in the friendly zone.

It is also a good time to mention—do not take on a parent-like role with Deaf students. Educational interpreters should not have relationships with Deaf students and their families outside of the school setting. Educational interpreters who babysit Deaf students on the weekend, drive them from school to after-school care, and/or take them to church on the weekend are fundamentally violating their role.

The *PIE Role Metaphor* for educational interpreters truly delineates the vast differences between interpreting for Deaf adults in community settings versus interpreting for Deaf students in a public-school setting. As educational interpreters, not only do we interpret, but we also prepare materials for interpretation, serve as a team liaison amongst many stakeholders, work as a consultant, advocate, and ally, all while simultaneously providing direct instruction, pre-teaching concepts, and being a helpful school system employee.

Movement between the various role positions on the "educational interpreting stage" is an autonomous professional decision (Fitzmaurice, 2017). The needs of the Deaf student and the context of the situation are always paramount in our decision-making process. On any given day, we may spend time interpreting, moving to being a helpful employee as the Deaf student is doing independent work, then being more personable as the Deaf student shares their weekend plans, then as a liaison sharing what happened during the lesson with the team, while also asking teachers what the next day's lesson will look like for us to prepare for interpreting, and for direct instruction to pre-teach vocabulary with the Deaf student. We are constantly moving between role areas within the larger educational interpreter role.

Counter to the *Davino Inverted Triangles of Responsibility* (above), there is absolutely no expectation that older students are going to need less social coaching, friendliness, or advocacy. Those absolutes are completely theoretical and vague. Such absolutes fail to consider how individual students become empowered and navigate the education system. However, if we are effective as educational interpreters early on, particularly with advocacy, we can and do transition into more of an ally.

General Interpreting Theories and Processes

Invariably, there are a multitude of interpreting theories, models, and processes ranging from cognitive models to textual models to interaction models and processing models (to categorize just a few) (Pöchhacker, 2016). Some models have firm roots in current interpreting practice. For example, interpreters are not simple machines (see the metaphors earlier in this chapter) but rather are directly involved in the interaction. Of course, there is a significant difference in interpreting practice when interpreting for adults versus children. We do not wish to address the multitude of interpreting and translation theories and models; rather, we share some that we find are helpful for educational interpreters.

Skopos Theory

In its original German origin, *skopostheorie* or *skopos theory* approaches translation acts (or, for our purposes, interpreting acts) as more functional and sociocultural leaning (Vermeer, 1989). *Skopos theory* suggests interpreting is not about a literal transcoding of words and propositions; rather, interpreting should be about calculating (and conveying) the purpose of the words. Instead of focusing on literal equivalence, *skopos theory* supports conveying meaning in a way that is culturally and linguistically appropriate for the audience. This means interpreters may adapt idioms, simplify language, or restructure messages to ensure the receiver understands the sender's intent. In educational settings, this is especially useful for ensuring Deaf students grasp the content and can engage meaningfully with instruction. This lens means we have met the fidelity rule in that the source message is coherent in the interpretation.

SF: One of my favorite examples is when a Deaf person refers to the state residential school by signing INSTITUTE. *This is problematic as, culturally, that has relevance to Deaf people but does not make much sense to hearing people. Interpreters rarely ever interpret that as "institute"; rather, they will often say "school," a linguistic choice that does not capture the cultural significance of the source. Considering skopos theory and dynamic equivalence, a more faithful interpretation must include a linguistic expansion such as "the state residential school for the Deaf" etc.*

Likewise, the English phrase "hold your horses" means be patient or wait. A literal (and ineffective interpretation) would look like: HOLD YOUR HORSE. This makes absolutely no sense in ASL since this rendition would refer to the physical animal being restrained or supported as opposed to the metaphorical meaning of the English expression. A better rendition that accounts for the overarching purpose of the communication would include the signs PATIENT or WAIT. This latter interpretation is faithful to the source message but accommodates for sociocultural and linguistic differences between both languages in line with the tenets of skopos theory.

This is key for educational interpreters in that often when Deaf students are learning to read, they are unaware of the idiomatic phrases they are reading and what they mean. Interpreters who work literally are simply ineffective. Dynamic equivalence wins every time against literal interpretation.

Gile's Effort Model

In the late 1980s, Daniel Gile introduced the *Effort Model* (Gile, 1988) as a conceptual framework to highlight the role of limited cognitive capacity in interpreting. He later expanded on this model to further explain the challenges interpreters face and how cognitive overload can lead to errors and omissions. At its core, the model suggests that when an interpreter devotes too much attention to comprehension, other essential cognitive tasks (such as production) may suffer.

Interpreting, by nature, demands significant mental resources, and when the required effort exceeds the available capacity (saturation), performance declines and the interpretation is prone to breakdowns. To better understand these demands, Gile (1992) categorized simultaneous interpreting tasks into four distinct but overlapping efforts: Listening and Analysis (reception), Memory (working memory), Production, and Coordination (SI=L+M+P+C). In later work, Gile (2009) emphasized that although sight translation, consecutive interpreting, and simultaneous interpreting involve different combinations of these efforts, they all draw from the same limited cognitive pool. Of course, there are contextual differences working in different settings (community, court, conference, remote, and, in this case, educational).

As a part of the *Effort Model*, Gile (2009) proposed the *Tightrope Hypothesis* which suggests interpreters often work close to cognitive saturation or capacity. Because interpreting is such a demanding cognitive task, unexpected things like having a fast speaker or signer or unfamiliar vocabulary can result in capacity overload and interpreting errors. More recently, Gile (2025) noted terminology in interpreting and translation has always been challenging and he has refined some of his terminology and clarified much of his work.

What is key is there are several strategies Gile offers to reduce the cognitive demands of interpreting. For example, using simpler sentence structures in the target language, omitting redundant information, using context to predict what the message may next be, and improving source language comprehension. For educational interpreters, this may look like more preparation with teaching materials, strategic omissions (Napier, 2004), and associating with Deaf adults as language models.

This overview of Gile's work is not exhaustive but serves to underscore just how cognitively demanding the task of interpreting truly is. Interpreting is not just about language transfer but about managing limited cognitive resources.

Cokely's Sociolinguistic Model of the Interpreting Process

Cokely's (1992) *Sociolinguistic Model of the Interpreting Process* was key to understanding interpreting as a discourse-based, interactional process (Pöchhacker, 2016) and not a word-for-word linguistic transfer. As a sociolinguistic model, Cokely highlighted the roles of culture, language variation, register, and interactional norms. Yet, it remains in use as a processing model in the field of interpreting, regardless of languages and cultures, with little direct sociolinguistic application. Cokely's model is complex but proposes seven essential processing stages:

1. Message reception: is the input good?
2. Preliminary processing: is the interpreter able to process this information?
3. Short-term memory retention: can the interpreter remember the key points?
4. Semantic intent realized: does the interpreter understand the content?
5. Semantic equivalence determined: has the interpreter figured out a faithful equivalent?
6. Syntactic message formulation: what are some factors to consider in this interpretation?
7. Message production: is the output good?

Once the first phrase of an interpretation has gone through this process, in simultaneous interpreting the process continually cycles through these seven stages.

Cokely (1992) also provided a taxonomy of miscues or errors which prove somewhat useful to analyze why a specific interpretation or text is challenging.

This is a holistically simplified explanation of Cokely's model, but we find it useful for educational interpreters to again think of it in terms of how complicated and demanding the act of interpreting is and, if an interpretation is ineffective, the means to determine where during the process the breakdown may have occurred. It is also important for educational interpreters to remember we are interpreting for children without solid language skills who are ultimately held accountable to demonstrate they understand the content.

Russell's Meaning-Based Model of Interpreting

Building on Cokely's model, Russell's (2002) *Meaning-Based Model of Interpreting* acknowledges the linguistic and cultural differences between two languages and cultures and is grounded in discourse analysis and constructivist views of interpreting.

Russell (2002) suggests interpreting encompasses meaning construction. Interpreting is not a sentence-by-sentence transfer but a process of constructing equivalent meaning in the target language. Meaning reconstruction must consider the sender's intent (skopos theory), the discourse context, and the cultural norms of both source and target communities. This means interpreters must focus on entire discourse events, not isolated utterances, particularly since meaning develops through interaction which requires interpreters to track cohesion, register, and pragmatics.

Interpreters must also monitor contextual influences (physical, social, and institutional contexts) along with the goals of participants, power dynamics, and setting norms—particularly in educational and legal environments.

Interpreters are encompassed as active participants in the discourse event (Roy, 2000; Wadensjö, 1998), viewed as co-participants and not as neutral channels. They make judgment calls about when to clarify or intervene. Interpreters are strongly encouraged to reflect on their decisions, analyze discourse interactions, and consider the ethical implications of their role and performance.

What is unique about Russell's model that is relevant to educational interpreters is the aspect of continually assessing the context. What does the Deaf student know about a topic already? Are there key terms the students need to know? What are students expected to know for testing purposes? Is the student looking at me or trying to find a page in the textbook? What do I as the educational interpreter know about this subject? Also, the educational interpreter is monitoring their process to ensure the Deaf student is understanding the interpretation, making adjustments or using repetition or rephrasing as necessary.

Later, Russell (2005) points to the opportunity to determine whether the interpreter would rather interpret consecutively or simultaneously.

Simultaneous interpreting tends to have more errors than consecutive interpreting due to the intense cognitive demands it places on the interpreter (Seeber & Kerzel, 2012). In simultaneous interpreting, the interpreter must listen, process, and render the message in the target language almost at the same time, leaving little opportunity to fully analyze or reformulate the message (Russell, 2005).

This constant multitasking relies heavily on short-term memory and can quickly lead to mental overload, especially with complex or fast-paced input (Cheung, 2024). Additionally, the interpreter has minimal time to correct mistakes or clarify misunderstandings, which increases the likelihood of omissions, distortions, or inaccuracies (Cox & Salaets, 2019). In contrast, consecutive interpreting allows interpreters to listen to longer segments of the source, take notes, and carefully reconstruct the message, resulting in fewer errors and a more accurate interpretation (Russell, 2005).

It is important for educational interpreters to know that most of our interpreting practices are simultaneous. However, in a classroom, there are ample opportunities to interpret consecutively; for example, one-on-one interactions with a teacher.

Overall, Russell's (2005) *Meaning-Based Model of Interpreting* shifts the focus from linguistic accuracy to communicative effectiveness, making it especially valuable in educational settings where meaning clarity and student inclusion are essential.

DC: I teach interpreting in a two-year program. For each text we interpret, I have my students do it consecutively first. Then we analyze the source, and THEN they interpret simultaneously. Many of them say that simultaneous is easier than consecutive, which is simply not true with respect to creating a cohesive interpretation. If you think simultaneous is easier, it is likely because you are concerned about "forgetting stuff," by which you mean words, which means your processing is at the lexical level and your interpretation is likely a "word salad." Instead, focus on the main ideas and reconstruct the message in the target language, centered around the main ideas.

Gish Model Applied to Educational Interpreting

One text analysis model we favor is the *Gish Construct for Interpreting: A Goal-to-Detail Model of Information Processing* (*Gish Model*) (Gish, 1987). The *Gish Model* is a top-down processing model emphasizing the macrostructure of a text. This affords interpreters (and interpreting students) a way to help analyze a text, understand its meaning as best we can as an interpreter, and make predictions of what may come next. Interpreters cannot catch every word or sign and will ultimately miss information while interpreting—particularly if the cognitive demand saturates the interpreter. In other words, the interpreter gets lost. The *Gish Model* does not consider power dynamics of the parties, or the cognition involved in interpreting and translation. However, we find the *Gish Model* to be a valuable way to analyze incoming information and maintain control over the interpretation. Plus, it helps us determine what to omit as needed. The model looks like the example in Figure 7.3.

Others have modified this model, visualizing it as an outline or another schematic. In Figure 7.4, we present this model as a PowerPoint slide.

Supported by practice with nuanced empirical foundations, Gish (1987) helps map out or contextualize what we should be doing as an interpreter in a teaching environment; but more importantly, this model makes it possible to analyze the efficacy of our interpretation and even predict what we may encounter.

For educational interpreters working with Deaf students, the *Gish Model* is very helpful when we may need to abandon some of the data and details and focus more on the Objectives or Units. For example, if an educational interpreter is able to grasp Objective A but no Units and just details, there is little for the Deaf student to connect together. Likewise, missing Objective B but catching Unit 2 would link Unit 2 to Objective A, creating a lot of confusion. See Figure 7.5, "an ineffective interpretation," for an idea of what this may look like.

Similarly, Figure 7.6 indicates an educational interpreter is only able to convey Objectives A and C, with a few Units and scattered Details, which will

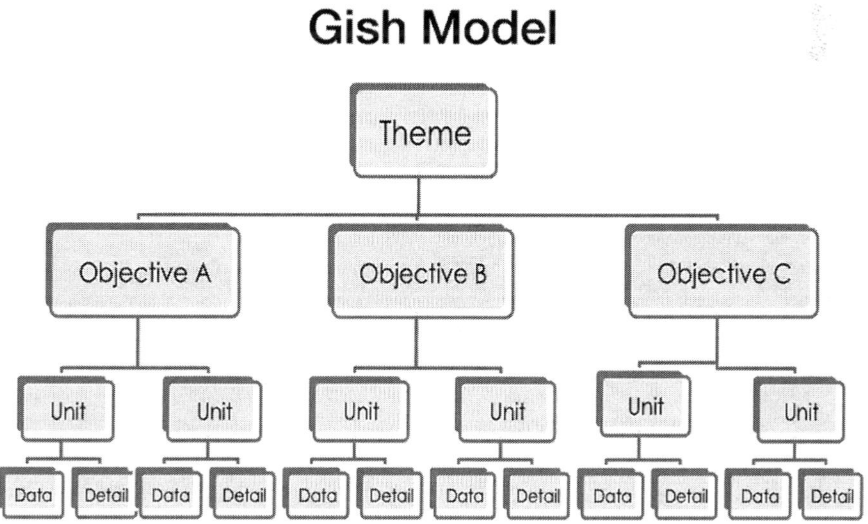

Figure 7.3 Gish Model

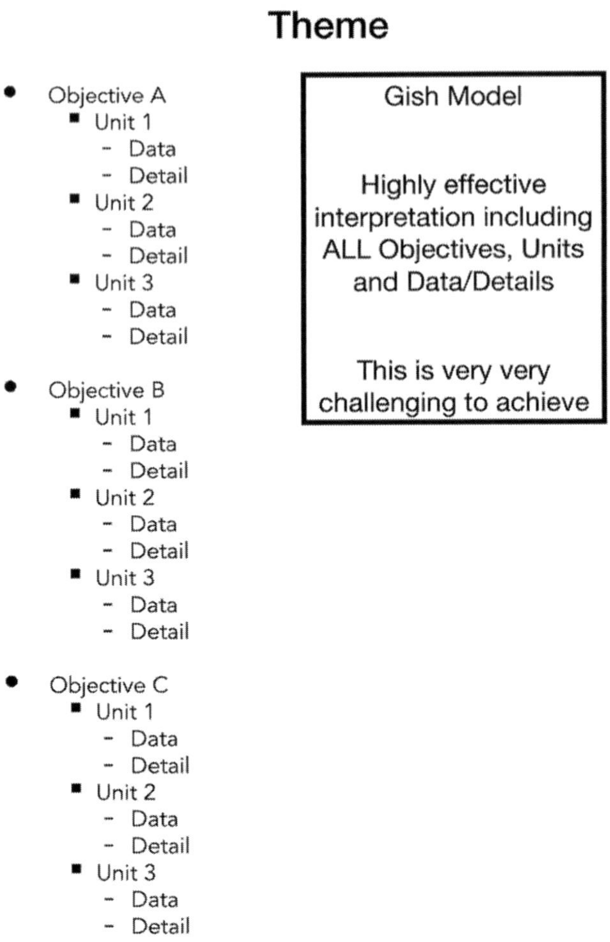

Theme

- Objective A
  - Unit 1
    - Data
    - Detail
  - Unit 2
    - Data
    - Detail
  - Unit 3
    - Data
    - Detail
- Objective B
  - Unit 1
    - Data
    - Detail
  - Unit 2
    - Data
    - Detail
  - Unit 3
    - Data
    - Detail
- Objective C
  - Unit 1
    - Data
    - Detail
  - Unit 2
    - Data
    - Detail
  - Unit 3
    - Data
    - Detail

Gish Model

Highly effective interpretation including ALL Objectives, Units and Data/Details

This is very very challenging to achieve

Figure 7.4 Gish Model as a PowerPoint Slide

invariably confuse the Deaf student, particularly if the student has language deprivation (see chapter five).

These types of interpretations happen as a result of educational interpreters focusing on words and details. It is almost impossible to catch every last detail, and attempting to do so ultimately results in getting lost conveying details but discursively not connecting them to anything. We strongly suggest educational interpreters whose work is characterized by disconnected data and details consider one of the two following approaches.

The first approach asks educational interpreters to forgo an entire Objective (in this case Objective B) and include Objective A and Objective C in their entirety while including all the Units and Data/Details. This is not ideal, but at least it provides a cohesive message to the Deaf student (see Figure 7.7).

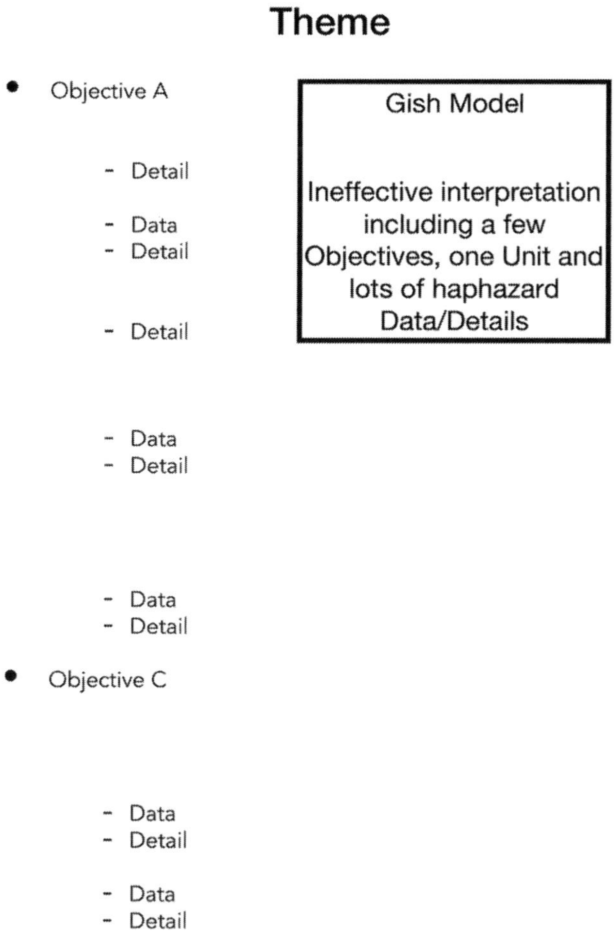

Figure 7.5 Ineffective interpretation A

The second and more effective approach means the educational interpreter does not worry about any of the data or details. Again, this is not ideal, but fundamentally the educational interpreter is at least able to convey all of the Objectives and Units—with a seamless link between those concepts. Figure 7.8 illustrates this approach.

Naturally, neither of these options are ideal as quite a bit of the source message is omitted, but if an educational interpreter is struggling with too much data and detail, we argue it is better to strategically discard some elements in order to ensure the portions we are able to include are cohesive and well-conveyed. An interpretation that has all of the data and details but none of the cohesion will be wholly incoherent to a Deaf student and will provide no educational benefit.

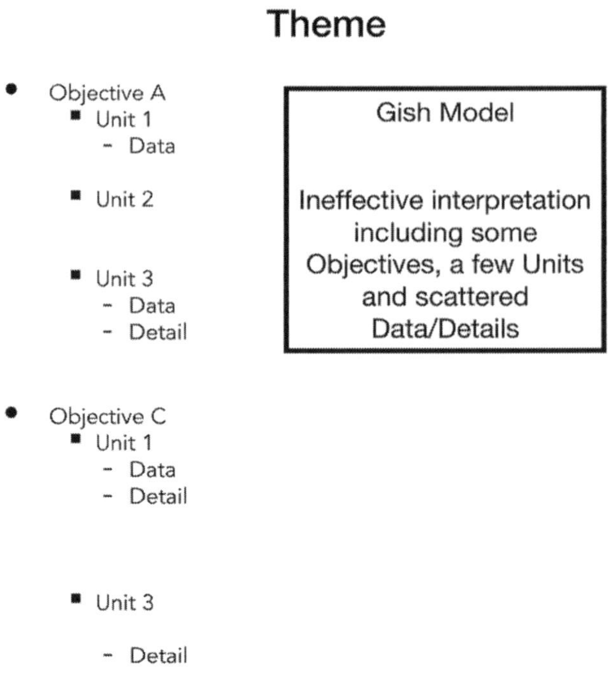

Figure 7.6 Ineffective interpretation B

DC: By way of illustration, there is a text I often use with my classes on the strengths and weaknesses of the Continental Army during the American Revolutionary War (explanatory text with a contrastive structure using comparative space). In this text, the teacher is contrasting the Continental Army's cause with the British Army's cause. The point she is making is that the Continental Army was fighting for a cause they believe in (family, home, freedom) whereas the British were ordered to fight. She says of the British, "They were told to get on a ship, cross the ocean, and stop this rebellion." In ASL, it takes time to set up the two countries, the ocean, the King ordering the troops, and the troops sailing across the ocean. This is data and detail. However, my students ALWAYS take the time to set up this visual at the expense of clearly interpreting the contrast between the two armies—that one army fought for a cause they were passionate about while the other army did not. It is better to include the contrast of having a cause versus not (Objective) and that one army was fighting for family, home, and freedom instead of being told they had to (Unit) and to drop the set-up of the army being ordered to cross the ocean (Detail) than to include the detail at the expense of the objective.

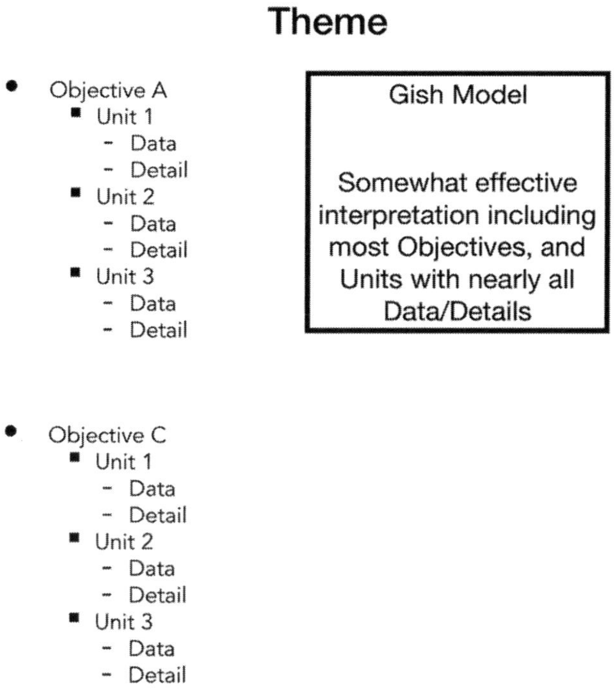

Figure 7.7 Somewhat effective interpretation

Strategic Omissions

Within any interpretation, there will be some omissions. Knowing and accepting that is part of our professional field. Napier (2004) has identified a taxonomy of omissions by interpreters. The first is a *conscious strategic omission* which is a deliberate omission in order to achieve a specific goal. *Conscious intentional omissions* are also deliberate omissions but without a specific strategy or goal involved. The third is a *conscious unintentional omission* which tends to happen because of an oversight on the interpreter's behalf. Omissions based on response or feedback from the student, though, are referred to as *conscious receptive omissions*. Lastly, *unconscious omissions* occur without the interpreter knowing about it. This frequently stems from an interpreter's lack of knowledge and/or a feeling of being overwhelmed.

Effective gaps (see Figure 7.8) employ *conscious strategic omissions* whereas ineffective gaps that cause a student to be confused are often the results of *conscious unintentional omissions* or *unconscious omissions* (see Figures 7.5 and 7.6). The educational interpreter is usually unaware that the resulting interpretation lacks cohesion and coherence.

In practical terms, we fully recognize that, as for any listener, we as educational interpreters can only infer what a teacher's Objectives and Units are. It is

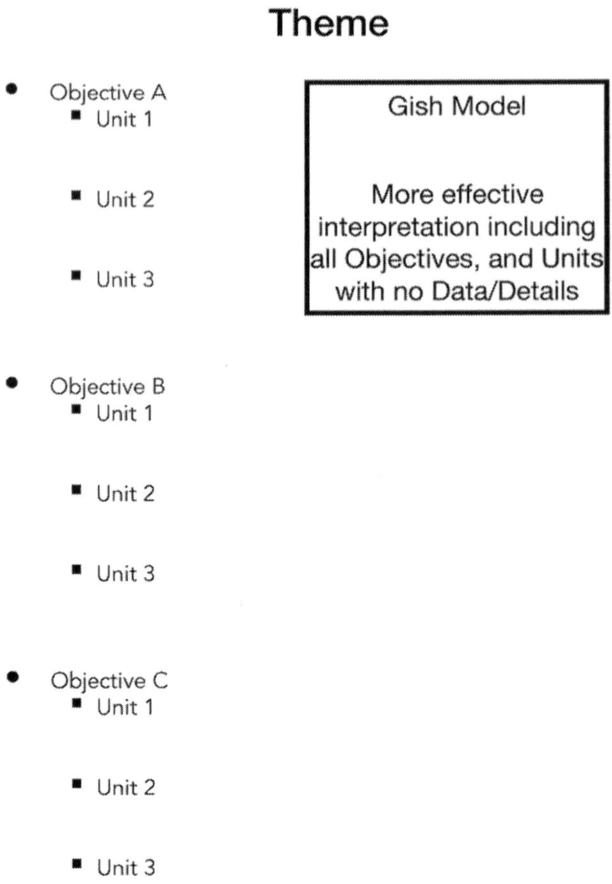

Figure 7.8 More effective interpretation

fairly easy to determine the general Theme by simply talking to a teacher beforehand about the lesson or major unit (theme) that the class will be discussing.

SF: I have found the best way to determine a teacher's objective is to simply ask (the day before): "For tomorrow's lesson, what takeaways do you want the students to know?" The answer tends to shed a lot of light on what the teacher (or curriculum) believes are the most important ideas. From there, data/details are also important to ask about. For example, "Are you wanting students to memorize key dates?" Again, talking with the team helps a lot.

DC: Note that there is a huge difference between asking about lesson takeaways and asking for lesson plans. Don't ask teachers for lesson plans. This is something their principals do to check up on them. According to a teacher friend of mine, her lesson plans are often messy and "just for her." She only drafts formal plans when a supervisor asks her to. So, do not ask for lesson plans. Focus on lesson takeaways and study the state standards for each subject in each grade instead.

Decision-Making: Beyond the Message

Dean and Pollard's Demand-Control Schema

Dean and Pollard's (2001) *Demand-Control Schema* (DCS) is a contextual framework for understanding the demands that are placed on an interpreter in a given situation, and the actions an interpreter can take to address those demands. it is not an ethical practices model, rather a decision-making tool that is informed by ethical principles (Dean & Pollard, 2011). The DCS has four different areas from which demands can stem: environmental, paralinguistic, interpersonal, and intrapersonal.

In educational settings, paralinguistic demands typically stem from either the student's language needs or from the need for the interpreter to have the language to discuss academic concepts in a variety of disciplines. Therefore, it is important for interpreters not just to study content information in English, but to find reputable Deaf teachers and study content taught in ASL. This goes far above and beyond simple vocabulary dictionaries. The Internet provides many opportunities for interpreters to study academic concepts being taught in ASL.

Many Deaf children in mainstream settings with an interpreter do not have access to ASL before working with an interpreter. Many working interpreters in education settings work with students that do not have a complete signed language before working with an interpreter (National Association of Interpreters in Education, 2019). Caselli, Hall, and Henner (2020) address this phenomenon of the illusion of inclusion. Many IEP Teams will place an educational interpreter with a student who has educational and language gaps with the assumption that the interpreter can fill both kinds of gaps. This is one of the reasons educational interpreters must be in constant contact with the child's IEP Team. They need to ensure that the team is aware of what the interpreter is seeing on a regular basis in the classroom. It is also critical for the interpreter to have an awareness of their own language, skills, and abilities, so they know what services they can and cannot provide.

Environmental demands as an educational interpreter often come from the classroom set-up. Mainstream classrooms are not designed to teach visual learners. They are designed around teaching auditory learners. Therefore, the interpreter may have to move around in order to be in the line of sight of the Deaf student. When teachers show videos in class and turn off the lights, the interpreter may need to ask to have the lights turned back on so the Deaf student can see them signing. Another environmental demand may come from the videos themselves if they do not have professional captioning, or if the child cannot read the captions. Once again, like with using educational interpreters, captions provide an illusion of inclusion when they may, in fact, not be accessible. We have addressed this point several times already, but it bears repeating because, in our experience, many interpreters fall into the trap of thinking captions provide access (see chapter five).

If captions are inaccurate, then the interpreter will need to interpret the video anyway. Even if the captions are accurate, the student may still benefit from seeing the video interpreted as prosodic information is lost in text (Jelinek Lewis & Jackson, 2001). The captions may also scroll too quickly for the student to read them, as we have discussed previously (Cambra, Silvestre, & Leal, 2009; Yoon & Kim, 2011). Another environmental demand in education comes from classroom noise. During group work, it is not uncommon for the classroom to be somewhat noisy, which may make it difficult for the interpreter to hear student conversation.

Interpersonal demands in educational settings often come from the dynamics between the interpreter and the classroom teacher. If a teacher has not worked with an interpreter before, the interpreter would benefit from some time to meet with the teacher before the start of the school year. Interpreters should be prepared to go into the classroom with an open mind and to engage in a dialogue with the teacher about their experiences with the Deaf child. Interpreters must remember that teachers are ultimately responsible for the entire classroom, including the Deaf student. Interpreters will sometimes mistakenly walk into a classroom with a set of demands to make of the teacher without knowing anything about the teacher's style, set-up, plans, background, knowledge, or goals. Ensure that your relationship with the classroom teacher gets off to a good start, as first impressions are lasting impressions.

Intrapersonal demands in educational settings may come from exhaustion due to long stretches of solo interpreting, isolation from other interpreting professionals, personal viewpoints that contradict what is being taught in any given class, and disagreements with IEP Team decisions.

DC: I am asthmatic. One day, an unexpected environmental demand caused me to have to leave the classroom. The teacher had sprayed air freshener in the room, and I had an asthma attack as a result.

Controls are the actions an interpreter can take to address demands. Controls are understood to be on a spectrum of conservative to liberal. Conservative controls are those that do not exercise a great deal of decision latitude (think *Conduit Metaphor*), whereas liberal controls do. For example, in the case of an environmental demand created by lighting, a liberal control would be the interpreter walking over to the light switch and adjusting the lighting in the room. A conservative control would be to ask the teacher to please turn on a light, or to wait until someone else notices that lighting is an issue.

Llewellyn-Jones and Lee's Role Space Model

Another way of understanding the scope of the interpreter's decision latitude is the *Role Space* model (Llewellyn-Jones & Lee, 2015), which challenges rigid definitions of an interpreter's role as fixed. In the *Role Space* model, the interpreter has latitude in their presentation of self, participant alignment, and interaction management. This latitude is constrained or expanded based on the characteristics of each unique situation.

Presentation of self is how much the interpreter represents themselves and their own thoughts in any given situation. Examples of presentation of self include introducing yourself using your first name or giving any kind of insight into your thoughts or feelings. It is common for educational interpreters to have a higher presentation of self than interpreters in community settings because educational interpreters work as a part of the educational team, and they see the same people every day.

DC: I like to use the example of people sharing about their weekend plans in preschool circle time versus at a board meeting. During preschool circle time, the interpreter will share about their weekend as the adults in the room take their turns sharing. They would NOT do so as the interpreter in a board meeting. If an interpreter behaved in preschool circle time the way they would in a board meeting, they would find themselves on the outs with that teacher.

Participant alignment is the degree to which an interpreter behaves more directly toward hearing participants or Deaf participants in a setting. Educational interpreters are often perceived as having much more Deaf participant alignment because they focus so much attention individually on Deaf students. However, interpreters working in classrooms with younger children may have broader alignment with hearing participants as well because they may provide support to hearing students in the classroom as well as to Deaf students. They may also need to explain aspects of their work to other children or adults in the setting.

Interaction management is a natural part of the interpreting process. The smaller the group of participants, the more of a role the interpreter plays in managing the interaction because participants will wait until an interpreter is done interpreting before taking their turn. This is not always the case. For example, in a setting where Deaf and hearing students are working together, hearing students may talk over one another and not give the interpreter an opportunity to interpret everything that is being said. In that case, interaction management would be the interpreter halting the conversation and asking students to take turns in order to allow them the opportunity to interpret everything. Interaction management may also happen when an interpreter interrupts a hearing person speaking in order to interpret what a Deaf person is signing. It is important to keep in mind that hearing people and Deaf people signal turn taking differently. When there is silence in a hearing person's conversation, that is a signal that it is time to turn over the floor. In other words, another speaker can step in and take their turn. However, in Deaf culture, eye gaze is the way turnover is managed. You know that it is your turn when your conversation partner looks at you, usually combined with dropping their hands and a head tilt or brow movement. Interpreters need to be aware of this as part of their function of interaction management.

DC: I was interpreting in a college class one time very early in my interpreting career, and there was a group discussion with multiple hearing students and one Deaf student. The Deaf student signed a remark pertinent to a piece of the conversation, but I was continuing to interpret what the hearing students were saying because there was no break in their conversation. By the time the Deaf student signed their comment during a pause where I could interpret it, the group had already moved on. I told the Deaf student that the hearing students had already moved on. I should not have done that. I have since learned how to politely interrupt when hearing people are talking in order to give voice to the Deaf person's comments. Hearing interpreters must always be aware that we are hearing people, and that we function with hearing cultural values and norms. Deliberate ethical practice includes learning and incorporating Deaf cultural values and norms.

Ethics

Ethics is an essential component of any practice profession. The CPC from the National Association of the Deaf and Registry of Interpreters for the Deaf (2005) is the default ethics document for the community interpreting profession. However, the National Association of Interpreters in Education (2021) has created the EICOE because educational interpreters are related service providers working under the auspices of a child's IEP. Educational interpreters are part of a team of professionals working to support the needs of a child, as well as working within an educational setting that has its own laws, practices, standards, and norms. This difference in role, responsibilities, and expectations creates a perceived conflict with the CPC, which was designed primarily with adult consumers in mind. Therefore, it was necessary to have a separate code of ethics for educational interpreters who are working with children (National Association of Interpreters in Education, 2021).

Confidentiality

Both codes of ethics contain statements of confidentiality. However, the educational interpreter is working as part of the educational team supporting a student. Therefore, they are asked to provide data about the Deaf student. These data may take the form of observations about how the student accesses their environment, information about what the child seems to understand or not understand with respect to language, how the child is using language within the classroom and to interact with peers, and any other relevant data related to the child's language or access to their environment. Likewise, both codes contain statements about the interpreter's role, but educational interpreters occupy a much larger role space than many interpreters working with adult consumers, as conceptualized in the *PIE Metaphor*.

Professional Development

Both the CPC and the EICOE include tenets about professional development. It is critical for any interpreter to engage in ongoing, robust professional development. This can be in the areas of skill development, enhancing knowledge, and preparation for assignments. As discussed above, interpreters in education are required to interpret an array of content. Students have core classes in math, science, English, and social studies. They also take classes in physical education and specials, such as art, music, STEM classes, and a variety of other coursework. This means that educational interpreters are required to know about a lot of different subjects. Professional development for educational interpreters should include studying content matter topics (in both ASL and English).

Respect for Consumers

Another area where the CPC and EICOE overlap is in the area of respect for consumers. In the case of the EICOE, interpreters are to respect student autonomy, which is explicitly stated in the EICOE since educational interpreters are working with minors. There is a tendency for interpreters to want to help, or to step in and do things for the student that the student can do on their own (enacting the *Helper Metaphor*). This is especially true for interpreters who follow one student from elementary to high school. Interpreters, like others in practice professions, have a tendency to have a "savior complex," wherein they feel the need to step in and "save" the Deaf student (Roy, 1993). Deaf students have the right to fail. They have the right to sleep through class. They have the right to ignore their interpreter. They have the right to blow off studying. They have the right to earn detention. Educational interpreters should get in the habit of checking themselves before intervening in any aspect of the Deaf student's education. First and foremost, the educational interpreter should ensure the student has the information they need to make an informed decision and then respect whatever decision they make. One practical way this plays out is when the Deaf student tunes out. Hearing students tune out all the time, but there are specific features of teacher speech that clue hearing students in to important information. Deaf students may not have access to these features of teacher speech, so interpreters should flag them and then let the Deaf student decide whether to tune back in or not.

The educational environment itself may result in situations where a student's autonomy is violated. For example, their IEP may state "preferential seating," which is often interpreted as sitting in the front of the classroom. However, not all students want to sit in the front of the classroom. They may prefer to sit off to the side where they can see their peers, or near the back of the room. When a Deaf student sits in the front of the room, they have a harder time accessing the conversations of their peers who are seated behind them. Another potential conflict between the educational environment and a student's autonomy is the requirement that the student wear their assistive listening devices or use frequency modulation (FM) systems, and so forth, at all times. Many Deaf students like to have breaks from the use of their hearing assistive technology. In some cases, the student may have a harder time focusing when they have their cochlear implants or hearing aids on. Interpreters should respect student choices and advocate with them to the IEP Team.

Respect for Colleagues

Both the CPC and EICOE contain statements of respect for colleagues. In the EICOE, this is expanded to include working with personnel in the educational environment. This includes teachers of the Deaf, speech language pathologists, and audiologists. Sometimes, other professionals on a student's educational team will have differing perspectives on best or effective practices for educating Deaf children. They may have differing perspectives on language for Deaf children, particularly when they view ASL as a communication tool. Educational interpreters must engage in respectful, but sometimes firm, dialogue with their colleagues.

Conduct

Perhaps one of the largest differences between the CPC and the EICOE is in the way they lay out expectations for interpreter conduct. While both codes contain guidance about avoiding conflicts of interest and avoiding dual roles, the conduct of an educational interpreter is going to differ substantially from that of an interpreter working with adult consumers because of the nature of the work. As discussed at length in this section, the roles educational interpreters inhabit include interpreting, team liaison, being a helpful employee, direct instruction, being an advocate, and being personable. For the most part, these functions are not considered appropriate conduct for an interpreter with adult consumers, and so many interpreters coming from a community setting feel at ethical odds with what is asked and expected of them in an educational setting.

Ethical Reasoning

Interpreters are often tempted to think of ethics as a set of rules for what is right and what is wrong. This is known as a *deontological approach*, which is aligned with the way the CPC was written and with a more *Conduit Metaphor* of interpreting. However, in the interpreting profession, ethical reasoning is shifting toward a more *teleological approach*. A teleological approach means that your focus is on the purpose served by whatever action you take (or don't take), rather than on a set of rules of right and wrong. A teleological approach is about how we use situational information plus our own values in order to determine ethically fit actions. As we have discussed above with DCS and Role Spaces, interpreters have different sets of controls, and situations allow for different degrees of latitude in exercising these controls. Therefore, an action that is considered "right" in one situation may be considered "wrong" in another situation (i.e., preschool classroom vs. boardroom), or with different consumers (i.e., native signer vs. student with language deprivation), or with a different interpreter (i.e., different controls). If we are choosing between what is absolutely right and what is absolutely wrong, we are using deontological reasoning. In order to understand the purpose served by any action in a given situation, interpreters have to understand the dynamics of the situation (DCS), they have to understand the participant roles and function of the interaction (Role Space), and they also have to understand values.

Values

Our values come from a variety of sources. We have personal values shaped by our own experiences and influenced by the environment we live in, by our families, our community, our faith, and our culture. For example, your socioeconomic class will influence how you perceive things like time, money, education, and socialization. You were not necessarily taught in any explicit way how to feel about these things, but the way that you were raised in your environment implicitly influenced and shaped your beliefs. Personal values are the root of our unconscious bias. As interpreters, ethical practice requires us to address unconscious bias, as it *will* affect how we interpret.

We also have values centered in our profession. We can find these values in the CPC and in the EICOE. Sometimes the values are stated explicitly, such as the core value statements with each tenet in the EICOE. Other times, values are implicit, such as the ordering of the tenets in both the CPC and EICOE. Ethical practice requires us to acknowledge these values and to examine the ways in which they influence our application of these codes to our practice.

In order to make ethical, impartial decisions, it is critical to identify the values at play in a given situation, the demands placed by the environment, the language needs of the consumers and setting, interpersonal, and intrapersonal factors, as well as understanding the nature of interaction dynamics in a given situation. When an interpreter has the opportunity to consider all of these things, they are then able to make a decision that is guided by values.

Here are some example scenarios from educational settings. For each of these scenarios, consider the demand(s), the possible control(s), the appropriateness of each control in the situation, the values involved, and potential outcomes from each control. Identify the tenet(s) from the CPC and EICOE implicated in each scenario. Identify where there is a value conflict and come up with potential solutions to address the conflict.

	Scenario
1.	You are interpreting for a Deaf student who uses cochlear implants. The student's IEP specifies that the child will wear their cochlear implant processors during all core classes. You notice that the child has started to remove their processors in some of their classes, especially during independent work time.
2.	You are interpreting in a middle school. The student to whom you are assigned has a couple of friends in the class who have been learning some conversational ASL. During the teacher's lecture, the student and their friends are having a conversation under their desks in ASL.
3.	You are asked to collect observational data about how the Deaf student is watching you during classes. You are asked to comment on how the child is functioning in their classrooms across the school day. This request is coming from a member of the child's IEP Team.
4.	You work for a school district that has multiple interpreters on the payroll. The interpreters take turns rotating out interpreting for different students in the district every school year. You are placed with a high school student who is taking several AP classes. One of the classes is AP calculus. You failed algebra in high school and never did calculus.
5.	You notice that the Deaf student with whom you work either gets up to sharpen their pencil or asks to use the restroom every single time that they are given an independent work task in a subject that is hard for them. You recognize that this is task avoidance behavior.
6.	You work with a student who uses comic book characters as their way of defining their relationships to others around them. The student casts themselves as the main character, and uses other characters such as villains, sidekicks, and love interests as their way of defining their relationship to other people. You notice that the student frequently assigns you the love interest character. You know from other interpreters who have worked with this student that interpreters are usually assigned a sidekick role.
7.	You are a male interpreter working with a female preteen student. The student wants to talk to her friends about having her period. You offer to interpret for the conversation and walk over with the student to her friends. She asks them if any of them have started their periods yet. Her friends just sit in silence and stare at you.
8.	You work at a high school. Hearing students in the classes where you interpret ask you to teach them swear words in ASL.
9.	You are asked to attend the IEP meeting for the student for whom you interpret. The student is also present at the meeting. You can tell by their expressions and responses that they do not understand the outside interpreter who was brought in to interpret the meeting.
10.	You live in a state that has separate requirements for interpreters working in education and interpreters working in the community. You are interpreting an evening sports activity when one of the students suffers an injury. They have to go to the hospital. You do not have the state credential in order to interpret in community settings, but the school district asks you to ride along to interpret for the injured student.

	Scenario
11.	You are interpreting, and the student asks you a question about one of the words that was said, but it is not a word that has any significance to the overall goal of the teacher's lecture.
12.	While you are interpreting for a teacher's lecture, a hearing student goes to get something from the counter, trips, bumps their face into the counter, and gets a bloody nose. You and the teacher are the only two adults in the classroom. The teacher asks you to walk the student to the nurse's office.

Summary

This chapter presented a comprehensive examination of the evolving role of educational interpreters, illustrating how simplistic metaphors like "Helper" or "Conduit" fail to capture the nuanced, multifaceted responsibilities these professionals carry in school settings. Through a critique of traditional metaphors and exploration of more dynamic frameworks—such as the Partners in Education (PIE) Role Metaphor—the chapter underscored the importance of recognizing educational interpreters as active, responsive members of the educational team. These interpreters must skillfully balance roles as language mediators, collaborators, instructional supporters, and advocates for student access and independence.

The chapter also integrated interpreting theories and models, such as Skopos Theory, Gile's Effort Model, Cokely's Sociolinguistic Model, and the Gish Model, which provide interpreters with tools for analyzing language use, managing cognitive demands, and ensuring meaningful communication. Additionally, frameworks like the DCS and Role Space help educational interpreters navigate the interpersonal, ethical, and contextual complexities of the classroom.

Ultimately, the chapter affirmed that effective educational interpreting requires more than technical skill—it demands preparation, ethical discernment, collaboration, and a deep commitment to student growth. By adopting student-centered approaches and leveraging evidence-based models, educational interpreters can create inclusive, empowering learning environments where Deaf students can thrive academically, socially, and linguistically.

Thought Questions

1 What is a conscious strategic omission versus an unconscious omission, and why might an interpreter use strategic omissions? How does the Gish Model help educational interpreters with strategic omissions?
2 How did the Conduit Metaphor arise as a response to the Helper Metaphor, and what are its limitations in interpreting?
3 What are the key responsibilities of educational interpreters as described through the Partners in Education (PIE) Role Metaphor?
4 What unique insights do interpreting theories and models offer to educational interpreters?

5 If an interpreter notices conflicting demands between classroom tasks and student needs, how can the Demand-Control Schema (DCS) guide their decision-making?
6 How does the Educational Interpreter Code of Ethics (EICOE) address the role of confidentiality differently from the NAD-RID Code of Professional Conduct (CPC)? Why is this distinction important in educational settings?

References

Antia, S. D., & Kreimeyer, K. H. (2001). The role of interpreters in inclusive classrooms. *American Annals of the Deaf*, 146(4), 355–365.

Baker-Shenk, C. (1991). The interpreter: Machine, advocate, or ally? In J. Plant-Moeller (Ed.), *Expanding horizons: Proceedings of the 1991 RID Convention* (pp. 120–140). Silver Spring, MD: RID Publications.

Cambra, C., Silvestre, N., & Leal, A. (2009). Comprehension of television messages by deaf students at various stages of education. *American Annals of the Deaf*, 153(5), 425–434.

Caselli, N. K., Hall, W. C., & Henner, J. (2020). American Sign Language interpreters in public schools: An illusion of inclusion that perpetuates language deprivation. *Maternal and Child Health Journal*, 24(11), 1323–1329.

Cheung, A. K. (2024). Cognitive load in remote simultaneous interpreting: Place name translation in two Mandarin variants. *Humanities and Social Sciences Communications*, 11: 1238.

Cokely, D. (1992). *Interpretation: A sociolinguistic model*. Burtonsville, MD: Linstok Press.

Cox, E., & Salaets, H. (2019). Accuracy: Omissions in consecutive versus simultaneous interpreting. *International Journal of Interpreter Education*, 11(2), 7–20.

Davidson, B. (2000). The interpreter as institutional gatekeeper: The socio-linguistic role of interpreters in Spanish-English medical discourse. *Journal of Sociolinguistics*, 4(3), 379–405.

Davino, D. (1985, February). The roles and responsibilities of the educational interpreter. Topic presented at the meeting of the Orange County Department of Education Secondary Hearing-Impaired Program staff, University High School, Irvine, CA.

Dean, R. K., & Pollard, R. Q. (2001). Application of demand-control theory to sign language interpreting: Implications for stress and interpreter training. *Journal of Deaf Studies and Deaf Education*, 6(1), 1–14.

Dean, R. K., & Pollard, R. Q. (2011). Context-based ethical reasoning in interpreting: A demand control schema perspective. *Interpreter and Translator Trainer*, 5(1), 155–182.

Fitzmaurice, S. (2017). Unregulated autonomy: Uncredentialed educational interpreters in rural schools. *American Annals of the Deaf*, 162(3), 253–264.

Fitzmaurice, S. (2021). *The role of the educational interpreter: Perceptions of administrators and teachers*. Washington, DC: Gallaudet University Press.

Gile, D. (1988). Le partage de l'attention et le "modèle d'efforts" en interprétation simultanée. *The Interpreters' Newsletter*, (1), 4–22.

Gile, D. (1992). Basic theoretical components in interpreter and translator training. In C. Dollerup & A. Loddegaard (Eds.), *Teaching translation and interpreting: Training, talent and experience* (pp. 185–193). Amsterdam: John Benjamins.

Gile, D. (2009). *Basic concepts and models for interpreter and translator training* (Rev. ed.). Amsterdam: John Benjamins.

Gile, D. (2025, March 20). The effort models and gravitational model: Clarifications and update [PowerPoint slides]. CIRIN. https://www.cirin-gile.fr/powerpoint/The-Effort-Models-and-Gravitational-Model-Clarifications-and-update.pdf.

Gish, S. (1987). I understood all the words, but I missed the point: A goal-to-detail/detail-to-goal strategy for text analysis. In M. McIntire (Ed.), *New dimensions in interpreter education: Curriculum and instruction* (pp. 125–137). Silver Spring, MD: RID Publications.

Jelinek Lewis, M. S., & Jackson, D. W. (2001). Television literacy: Comprehension of program content using closed captions for the deaf. *Journal of Deaf Studies and Deaf Education*, 6(1), 43–53.

Lawson, H. R., & Hamrick, M. (2011). Distribution of responsibilities.

Lee, R. G., Winston, E. A., & Forestal, E. M. (2023). Lessons from American Sign Language–English interpreting. *PMLA*, 138(3), 833–837.

Llewellyn-Jones, P., & Lee, R. G. (2015). *Redefining the role of the community interpreter: The concept of role-space*. Duluth, MN: Digiterp Communications.

Metzger, M. (1995). *The paradox of neutrality: A comparison of interpreters' goals with the reality of interactive discourse* (Unpublished doctoral dissertation). Georgetown University, Washington, DC.

Napier, J. (2004). Interpreting omissions: A new perspective. *Interpreting*, 6(2), 117–142.

National Association of Interpreters in Education. (2019). Professional guidelines for interpreting in educational settings (1st ed.). www.naiedu.org/guidelines.

National Association of Interpreters in Education. (2021). Educational interpreter code of ethics. https://naiedu.org/codeofethics/.

National Association of the Deaf & Registry of Interpreters for the Deaf. (2005). Code of professional conduct. Arlington, VA: Registry of Interpreters for the Deaf, Inc. https://rid.org/programs/ethics/code-of-professional-conduct/.

Pöchhacker, F. (2016). *Introducing interpreting studies* (2nd ed.). London: Routledge.

Roy, C. B. (1993). The problem with definitions, descriptions, and the role metaphors of interpreters. *Journal of Interpretation*, 6(1), 127–154.

Roy, C. B. (2000). *Interpreting as a discourse process*. New York: Oxford University Press.

Russell, D. (2002). *Interpreting in legal contexts: Consecutive and simultaneous interpreting*. Burtonsville, MD: Linstok Press.

Russell, D. (2005). Consecutive and simultaneous interpreting. In T. Janzen (Ed.), *Topics in signed language interpreting: Theory and practice* (pp. 135–164). Amsterdam: John Benjamins.

Seeber, K. G., & Kerzel, D. (2012). Cognitive load in simultaneous interpreting: Model meets data. *International Journal of Bilingualism*, 16(2), 228–242.

Smith, M. B. (2013). *More than meets the eye: Revealing the complexities of an interpreted education*. Washington, DC: Gallaudet University Press.

Tiselius, E., & Englund Dimitrova, B. (2023). Monitoring in dialogue interpreting: Cognitive and didactic perspectives. In L. Gavioli & C. Wadensjö (Eds.), *The Routledge handbook of public service interpreting* (pp. 309–324). London: Routledge.

Vermeer, H. J. (1989). Skopos and commission in translational action. In A. Chesterman (Ed.), *Readings in translation theory* (pp. 173–187). Helsinki: Oy Finn Lectura Ab. (Original work published 1984).

Wadensjö, C. (1998). *Interpreting as interaction*. London: Longman.

Yoon, J., & Kim, M. (2011). The effects of captions on deaf students' content comprehension, cognitive load, and motivation in online learning. *American Annals of the Deaf*, 156(3), 283–289.

8 Logistics of Educational Interpreting

Educational interpreting is a complex and demanding profession that requires a unique combination of cognitive skills and personal qualities. Interpreters must swiftly navigate linguistic challenges while managing the emotional pressures of supporting Deaf students in educational settings. Success in this field hinges not only on mental agility and extensive knowledge but also on personality traits such as resilience, empathy, and emotional stability. This chapter explores the multifaceted nature of educational interpreting, covering cognitive and emotional demands, performance assessments, certification standards, job logistics, professional development, classroom dynamics, and strategies for maintaining physical and emotional well-being. Understanding these interconnected elements is essential for interpreters to effectively support Deaf students and sustain long-term careers in education.

Personality Aspects

Personality is a mix of values, temperament, coping strategies, and motivation, and can incorporate other cognitive and social factors. A personality trait is how you as a person think or how you tend to do things in a variety of situations. Both general cognitive abilities and personality factors influence how people interact and manage their world experiences. Some researchers refer to general cognitive abilities as "can do" ingredients, such as the capacity to do the job. Personality aspects are sometimes referred to as the "will do" ingredients, such as dependability, motivation, confidence, or flexibility (Campbell, McCloy, Oppler, & Sager, 1993; Tett & Burnett, 2003). In other words, we manage our experiences through a blend of capacity and willingness.

In the interpreting field, cognitive capacity plays an important role (Gile, 2009; Macnamara, 2009; Pöchhacker, 2016). Interpreting simultaneously in two different modalities is undoubtedly a demanding task, which is further complicated by a diverse range of speakers and signers with whom you will interact (Macnamara, Moore, Kegl, & Conway, 2011; 2014). In addition, the fact that Deaf students often do not have a fully formed language makes the task all the more challenging. Interpreting requires extensive cognitive resources and brain horsepower, including among others, extensive reasoning ability, quick

DOI: 10.4324/9781003423058-8

thinking, higher-order thinking, substantial mental flexibility, rapid task switching, and robust working memory.

Personality aspects also account for specific aptitudes that apply to our work as educational interpreters. Researchers find successful interpreters tend to be highly self-confident, emotionally stable, able to use positive coping resources, open to experiences, have high levels of conscientiousness, and tend to favor extroversion (Shaw & Hughes, 2006). Interpreter educators also work to promote higher-order thinking skills and develop self-confidence in their students (Bontempo & Napier, 2007; Fitzmaurice, 2010).

The emotional stability continuum is a psychological spectrum that describes how individuals manage their emotions, particularly under stress or pressure (McCrae & Costa, 1999). On one end of the continuum are individuals who are emotionally reactive, prone to anxiety, and less resilient in the face of challenges. On the other end are those who demonstrate calmness, resilience, adaptability, and the ability to recover quickly from stressful experiences. This continuum is especially relevant in the context of interpreting, where practitioners regularly encounter high-pressure situations, rapid decision-making, and emotionally charged content. Research suggests that successful interpreters tend to fall on the emotionally stable end of the continuum. They exhibit high self-esteem, emotional resilience, openness to new experiences, and a strong sense of conscientiousness. These traits not only contribute to an interpreter's capacity to manage stress effectively, but also support their ability to remain present, think critically, and make ethical decisions in complex environments. Notably, many of these characteristics are interconnected with self-confidence and effective stress management—two essential components of interpreter readiness and professional longevity. Thus, emotional stability is not merely a personality trait but a foundational element of professional competence in the interpreting field.

One of the emotional stability continuum factors is conscientiousness. As a construct for interpreters, conscientiousness includes traits such as being self-disciplined, dependable, goal-oriented, efficient, and/or a perfectionist (though perfection is nearly impossible in our field) (Horváth, 2011). Most interpreters tend to be assertive, resourceful, confident, and stress resistant, rather than being overly rigid, unreliable, or having low self-confidence (Yang, 2025).

Common descriptors of educational interpreters often reflect personality profiles characterized by qualities such as being amiable, flexible, patient, relaxed, resilient, self-confident, self-motivated, steady, a team player, and understanding. These traits not only support the demanding cognitive and linguistic aspects of interpreting but also contribute to maintaining positive interpersonal relationships within educational environments. Interpreters frequently operate in dynamic and unpredictable settings, requiring them to remain calm under pressure, adapt to changing classroom dynamics, and respond empathetically to the needs of diverse students and team members.

Moreover, several of these characteristics—particularly patience, dependability, and empathy—are directly linked to effective teamwork. Being a dependable team player ensures consistency and trust within interdisciplinary teams that may include teachers, therapists, and school administrators (Witter-Merithew & Johnson, 2005). Patience allows interpreters to navigate developmental and language acquisition delays with grace and persistence, especially when working with Deaf students who have additional disabilities or who come from linguistically diverse backgrounds. Empathy, a cornerstone of both interpersonal communication and ethical practice, enables interpreters to consider the perspectives of others and respond in ways that foster collaboration and student-centered support.

Taken together, these personality traits create a profile of interpreters who are not only linguistically competent but also socially and emotionally attuned—qualities essential for building inclusive, supportive, and effective educational environments.

In the specific context of educational interpreting, these personality traits become even more critical. Educational interpreters work in dynamic, high-stakes environments that demand not only linguistic competence but also emotional resilience, ethical decision-making, and the ability to collaborate within interdisciplinary teams.

We share this information not to suggest that only individuals with a fixed personality profile can succeed in educational interpreting, but rather to support emerging interpreters in thoughtful self-reflection. Interpreting—particularly in educational settings—is not universally suited to every personality type. The profession requires a tolerance for ambiguity, a deep well of patience, and a genuine commitment to student development and access. For this reason, understanding one's strengths, challenges, and natural dispositions can help determine whether this career path is a good fit. Moreover, identifying the personal characteristics most relevant to interpreter success may guide professional development goals, helping individuals build the skills and emotional capacities needed to thrive in the field over time (Witter-Merithew & Johnson, 2005; Bontempo & Napier, 2007).

In essence, personality is not a fixed barrier or gatekeeper to entering the profession, but rather a useful lens for assessing readiness and identifying growth areas that will support long-term success and well-being as an educational interpreter.

Extralinguistic Knowledge (ELK)

Extralinguistic knowledge (ELK) refers to everything you know that is not specifically related to language. Every experience that you have ever had in your life contributes to your ELK. ELK affects your processing (Gile, 2025). If you understand the topic you are interpreting, you do not need as much *Listening and Analysis Effort* to process the information. If you do not know the content, you may require additional time, thereby leaving less capacity for *Production Effort* and *Coordination Effort*. Overall, the more effortful your process, the longer processing time you will require.

In general, interpreters often make the mistake of keeping very close to the speaker or signer if they are interpreting information with which they are unfamiliar, because they are afraid of making omissions (Angelelli, 2004; Napier, 2004; Napier, McKee, & Goswell, 2006). If an educational interpreter has some ELK on the topic, they will be less likely to begin interpreting too closely to the teacher's utterance, which reduces the number of omissions. The same is true when interpreting for someone who speaks or signs very rapidly. However, this tendency of keeping very close to the speaker or signer can lead to a less *cohesive* interpretation because the interpreter is not taking the necessary time to analyze the source for meaning. While increased processing time results in more opportunity for *strategic omissions* (Angelelli, 2004; Napier 2004), the end product will be more *cohesive* and likely will reflect more of the main ideas from the source.

Again, the more ELK you have or "the more stuff you know about things," the less cognitive stress you will experience (Gile, 2025). Although ELK does not make up for a lack of requisite language skills, it does allow you to maximize them.

This is one of the reasons a well-rounded general education is essential for educational interpreters. If you have a hobby, everything that you have learned associated with that hobby is ELK. If there are specific subjects that you have studied with any kind of intent, they are part of your ELK. An interpreter's ELK is one of their most valuable assets.

As an educational interpreter, you do not have the luxury of accepting or declining assignments on the basis of content the way community freelancers can. Like Video Relay Service (VRS) interpreters, educational interpreters cover every subject throughout their careers. Therefore, any additional learning that you can do on any topic is going to be beneficial to you in the classroom. Fortunately, unlike VRS interpreters, educational interpreters have some idea of what the student will be learning over the course of an academic year because of the structured *curriculum*.

Developing ELK goes far beyond just learning signs or vocabulary for specific concepts; interpreters need to understand these concepts as a system and the relationships between ideas within the system. Interpreters frequently seek out vocabulary workshops in order to address gaps in their language proficiency. These workshops can be useful; however, they may not provide as much information about how the vocabulary is used and understood in context. Content-specific workshops that present vocabulary in its broader context within the subject matter will be far more effective for building ELK than vocabulary-specific workshops. American Sign Language (ASL) discourse features (e.g., faceting, explained by examples, contrasting, use of 3-D space, reiterating, scaffolding, and "describe then do") can be used to express concepts in ASL if there is not a standard lexical sign (Janzen, 2005; Valli, Lucas, Mulrooney, & Villaneuva, 2011; Wilcox, 2000). Remember, ASL is a compounding language! However, in order to be able to appropriately deploy these discourse features, you will need to understand the concepts about which you are interpreting.

There are *core standards* available for interpreters to reference for each topic and grade level. If there is a school subject with which you are unfamiliar, it is important for you to develop your ELK in that area. It may be beneficial for you to study a topic with which you are unfamiliar during professional development time. In addition to course materials, there are also a variety of online resources available to you for developing ELK and to help prepare for class. Consider searching for video tutorials on a variety of subjects that are scaffolded by topic or grade level. There are also several excellent online resources for academic ASL, and of course reading extensively across a range of topics is always valuable. Again, the more you know, the more you expand your ELK, which can reduce the cognitive load of interpreting.

The Educational Interpreter Performance Assessment (EIPA)

The Educational Interpreter Performance Assessment (EIPA) is the most well recognized nationwide assessment for educational interpreters, developed in 1991 by Schick and Williams. The EIPA is designed to assess features that interpretations must have specifically in educational settings, and therefore places emphasis on areas such as prosody, fingerspelling, and the organization of information in an interpretation. There is a written portion and a skills portion.

EIPA Written Test (EIPA:WT)

The EIPA written test (EIPA:WT) is designed to assess the knowledge, ethics, and practices of interpreters working in educational settings. There are nine domains on the EIPA:WT. These domains include linguistics, child language development, technology, literacy and tutoring, education, English, culture, interpreting, and professionalism.

The test consists of 176 questions, and it is a pass/fail test. For more information on the written test, including access to the standards from which the written test was developed, please see www.classroominterpreting.org.

Your coursework in educational interpreting is an excellent way to prepare for the EIPA:WT. This textbook has also been designed to support novice interpreters to prepare for the test by covering a broad range of the topics covered on the exam.

Unlike community-based interpreting exams, the EIPA:WT is not required prior to taking the performance assessment. Some states require interpreters to take the written test, and other states do not.

EIPA Performance Test

Educational interpreters choose between interpreting stimulus materials using ASL or Contact Sign (PSE) and then select materials at the elementary or secondary level. There are several lessons in each version of the test, and educational interpreters are provided preparation material for each classroom vignette. Educational interpreters also select one of two child signers to interpret from ASL or Contact Sign (PSE) into English.

There are 37 individual skill indices that are each rated from 0 to 5 on a Likert-type scale. These 37 indices are broken down into four domains (the Romans):

- Roman I measures an interpreter's ability to interpret from English into ASL or Contact Sign (PSE) with 11 indices across four sub-categories: prosodic information, non-manual information, use of space, and grammatical information (interpreter performance).
- Roman II measures an interpreter's ability to interpret from ASL or Contact Sign (PSE) into English, with ten indices across four sub-categories: reading/conveying the signer's intent and content, vocal and intonational features, word choice, and absence of extraneous sounds/words.
- Roman III measures an interpreter's overall vocabulary skills with nine indices across two sub-categories: signs and fingerspelling.
- Roman IV measures the features of an interpretation that give an overall representation of the equivalency between source and target messages. There are seven indices in this domain, five of which deal with expressive skills and two with receptive skills. The three sub-categories in this domain are message processing, message clarity, and environmental information.

Scores within each Roman are averaged together to give individual Roman scores, and those are then averaged together for the overall score.

In addition to receiving individual scores on each index, interpreters receive comments on their areas of strength and areas of need. The initial page of the report gives an overall snapshot of the interpreter's strengths and weaknesses, and then, in each individual Roman, they receive feedback on areas of strength and areas of weakness.

There are scoring patterns on the EIPA. Most educational interpreters score highest in Roman III, the vocabulary domain. Roman I is the next highest scoring domain, followed by Roman II, and then Roman IV. For a detailed breakdown of the score patterns, see Cates (2021). Generally, score patterns indicate that interpreters tend to be able to interpret words and sentences with relative ease (bottom-up) but struggle to represent features of higher-level discourse (top-down). This reflects what we have discussed previously in this book about interpreter processing—it is more than just using signs for words and words for signs. However, many interpreters do not receive sufficient training in how to process information in a top-down way before attempting to take the EIPA. Therefore, as you are learning how to interpret, focus on the goal and main ideas of the source message as an intentional exercise. Develop your ability to summarize information and to identify main ideas and key details. Get into the habit of assessing information for its relationship to the goal and main ideas while you are interpreting.

Table 8.1. EIPA levels. Table 8.1 details the descriptions of an interpreter's skill at each level (Educational Interpreter Performance Assessment, n.d.; National Consortium of Interpreter

Level 1: Beginner:	Demonstrates very limited sign vocabulary with frequent errors in production. At times, production may be incomprehensible. Grammatical structure tends to be non-existent. Individuals are only able to communicate very simple ideas and demonstrate great difficulty comprehending signed communication. Sign production lacks prosody and use of space for the vast majority of the interpreted message. An individual at this level is not recommended for classroom interpreting.
Level 2: Advanced Beginner:	Demonstrates only basic sign vocabulary and these limitations interfere with communication. Lack of fluency and sign production errors are typical and often interfere with communication. The interpreter often hesitates in signing, as if searching for vocabulary. Frequent errors in grammar are apparent, although basic signed sentences appear intact. More complex grammatical structures are typically difficult. Individual is able to read signs at the word level and simple sentence level, but complete or complex sentences often require repetitions and repairs. Some use of prosody and space, but use is inconsistent and often incorrect. An individual at this level is not recommended for classroom interpreting.
Level 3: Intermediate:	Demonstrates knowledge of basic vocabulary, but may lack vocabulary for more technical, complex, or academic topics. Individual is able to sign in a fairly fluent manner using some consistent prosody, but pacing is still slow with infrequent pauses for vocabulary or complex structures. Sign production may show some errors but generally will not interfere with communication. Grammatical production may still be incorrect, especially for complex structures, but is in general, intact for routine and simple language. Comprehends signed messages but may need repetition and assistance. Voiced translation often lacks depth and subtleties of the original message. An individual at this level would be able to communicate very basic classroom content but may incorrectly interpret complex information, resulting in a message that is not always clear. An interpreter at this level needs continued supervision and should be required to participate in continuing education in interpreting.
Level 4: Advanced Intermediate:	Demonstrates broad use of vocabulary with sign production generally correct. Demonstrates good strategies for conveying information when a specific sign is not in their vocabulary. Grammatical constructions are generally clear and consistent, but complex information may still pose occasional problems. Prosody is good, with appropriate facial expression most of the time. May still have difficulty with the use of facial expression in complex sentences and adverbial non-manual markers. Fluency may deteriorate when rate or complexity of communication increases. Uses space consistently most of the time, but complex constructions or extended use of discourse cohesion may still pose problems. Comprehension of most signed messages at a normal rate is good but may lack some complexity of the original message. An individual at this level would be able to convey much of the classroom content but may have difficulty with complex topics or rapid turn-taking.

Level 5: Advanced:	Demonstrates broad and fluent use of vocabulary, with a broad range of strategies for communicating new words and concepts. Sign production errors are minimal and never interfere with comprehension. Prosody is correct for grammatical, non-manual markers, and affective purposes. Complex grammatical constructions are typically not a problem. Comprehension of signed messages is very good, communicating all details of the original message. An individual at this level is capable of clearly and accurately conveying the majority of interactions within the classroom.

State Requirements

As a diagnostic assessment, the EIPA performance assessment does not have pass/fail scoring. Many states, however, use the overall EIPA score to establish minimum competency standards. The National Association of Interpreters in Education (NAIE) (2023) maintains a map of information on specific state requirements. In their *Professional Guidelines for Interpreting in Educational Settings* (NAIE, n.d.), the NAIE also recommends educational interpreters have an EIPA score of 4.0 or higher, a passing score on the EIPA:WT, and a bachelor's degree in interpreting.

From 2007 to 2016, the RID offered the Ed:K-12 national certification for members who earned over an EIPA 4.0, passed the EIPA:WT, and held a baccalaureate degree. However, that certification is in moratorium and unlikely to be offered again in the future (ASL Interpreting, n.d.). At the time of this writing, there is no certifying body for the EIPA; therefore, one cannot be "EIPA certified." However, at the time of this writing, the NAIE is currently exploring the development of a nationally recognized certification system specifically for educational interpreters.

Generally, states manage the minimum competency expectations for educational interpreters using one of three approaches. The first is state licensure, which is typically the product of a state statute outlining the licensing requirements for educational interpreters and tends to be more heavily enforceable. The second approach is regulation, generally developed by the State Board of Education, that outlines the qualifications needed in order to work for a school system. This approach is binding but not always enforced. The final approach is state guidelines or guidance documents. These are neither binding nor enforceable. Educational interpreters can find information about state requirements through the NAIE website.

We note that many states have a minimum competency at or below an EIPA 3.5. The EIPA Diagnostic Center indicates an educational interpreter with an EIPA score less than 4.0 requires supervision. This is borne out by research indicating educational interpreters with an EIPA 3.0 do not provide educational benefit to students (Cates & Delkamiller, 2021) but that educational interpreters with an EIPA 4.0 provide roughly the same educational benefit as an instructor who uses simultaneous communication. Again, research repeatedly shows that even the most highly qualified educational interpreter cannot provide the same educational benefit as a fluent teacher of the Deaf (TOD) providing direct instruction in ASL.

Before You Begin

Logistics

There are several considerations to make before applying for a job as an educational interpreter. In this section, we will cover hiring practices, interview questions to ask, placements, supervision, working environment, scheduling, and professional development.

Hiring Practices

There are different ways to become an educational interpreter. Each path brings with it different considerations and questions you should ask in the process of applying for a position. The most common way is to be hired directly by a school district. School districts may hire a single interpreter for a single Deaf student, or they may employ multiple interpreters to serve a larger population of Deaf students. Both of those situations are going to result in different considerations.

If you are going to be working for a school district with a single student, you will want to request support from the school district going into the position with professional development opportunities, specific training opportunities for aspects of your job in which you have not been trained, and opportunities to network with other educational interpreters. You will also want to learn as much about the student as possible to make sure you are a good fit. Often, these positions for a single interpreter for a single student occur in small, rural school districts where there is not as much community support. There is also not as much funding for additional positions and support for Deaf students, so more responsibilities are likely to fall to the educational interpreter.

When working for a school district that employs a group of interpreters, ask about their practices regarding placing interpreters with students. Ask if you will have an opportunity to team with other interpreters, or if you will be expected to work by yourself all day long. Ask if there is an opportunity for interpreters to switch assignments during the day in order that each interpreter working for the district can cover the topics they are most familiar with. Also, inquire if you can work with other students or if you will be assigned to a single student all day every day.

Another way you may be hired to work as an educational interpreter is through a regional education program. These programs have different names, but they function as a state-run agency that provides special education (SPED) support to school districts. These regional programs may employ a cadre of interpreters who are then assigned to school districts as those districts have need. In such a case, you may work in different schools over a larger area, you may work by yourself, or you may work with others in the same building. If you are hired in this situation and other interpreters work for the same regional program, inquire about opportunities for professional development or collaboration with the other interpreters that work for the same regional program.

Another way you may work for a school district is by placement through an interpreting agency. Interpreting agencies may have contracts with school districts to provide their educational interpreter services on an ongoing basis, or they may provide interpreters when school districts cannot fill open positions. In a situation like this, you may work with one student all day every day for a school year, or you may only work certain days of the week with that student. You may also simply sub occasionally in schools. If you are working for a school district through an agency, the information you receive about the position will come through the agency initially, not from the school district. Many agency-employed interpreters work primarily in community settings, so agencies do not ask the same types of questions that you would ask before working with a school district. If you plan to work for an interpreting agency and to accept jobs in education, give them a list of questions you would like them to ask of a school district to aid you in determining whether it is ethical for you to accept the assignment.

Questions to Ask

Here are some questions to consider before you apply for a job, questions to ask in an interview, or questions to ask of an agency before they place you with a student. Ask about student language use. As we have discussed in this book, students have a variety of needs regarding their language. Some will use spoken English receptively and expressively with ASL as a visual support to fill in gaps or clarify hard-to-distinguish words, some will use only ASL expressively and receptively, and many students will use a combination of both. It is important to know what type of language access the student requires so you know if you have the appropriate level of fluency. Ask about the student's age, grade level, and placement. The younger the student is, the more time you will spend doing direct instruction. Their grade level will tell you something about the types of classes they may be taking. If you can see a copy of the student's schedule, that is even better because it will tell you more about their placement—i.e., how much time is spent in a resource or self-contained room versus the general education classroom. Ask about any additional identified needs they may have. Ask what previous service providers have done with the student besides interpreting. Ask specifically about behavior interventions, toileting and other personal hygiene, and the need for the student to have an interpreter with them at recess and lunch. Find out when you have scheduled breaks and lunch, especially if the student needs an interpreter with them during recess and lunch times.

Another important aspect of considering a job as an educational interpreter is the job description. Review it carefully. Educational interpreter job descriptions vary depending on how the school district has classified the position. School districts that have classified educational interpreters with paraprofessionals will have more in their job description about supporting students with things like behavior, instructional materials, toileting, and other types of non-interpreting-related duties. Every school district will have a phrase in their job description that says, "other duties as assigned." This is included in job descriptions as a catch-all to allow school districts to ask you to do things without having to delineate every duty that may come up. Other duties as assigned typically include room monitoring, recess or lunch duty, doing morning or afternoon bus duty, or other small tasks such as making copies or assisting teachers with preparing materials for their classroom. Ask what the school expects of you regarding these other duties.

We have covered the *Partners in Education (PIE) Metaphor* for educational interpreters in chapter seven. The PIE Metaphor gives you several responsibilities that are common to an educational interpreter role (Fitzmaurice, 2021a). The PIE Metaphor can help you in understanding and talking about how much time you spend on a given task area. You can also use the job description in order to help you figure out how well the district description aligns with your interpreting role. When job classifications are created, it is common for them to be based upon the expectation of what percentages of time will be spent in a particular duty or responsibility. The PIE Metaphor can help you to delineate the types of responsibilities that you may have as an educational interpreter, and help you to understand how those percentages are likely to change, depending on where you are placed.

Placement

It is important to understand the type of placement the student is in so you have some idea of what your role and responsibilities will look like. These responsibilities include advocating, providing direct instruction, being a helpful employee, being a team liaison, and interpreting. While any educational interpreter will spend at least part of their time engaging in each of these responsibilities, the time spent in each area will change depending on a lot of factors, including placement.

The amount of direct instruction you do will vary. Remember that the more time that you as an interpreter spend doing direct instruction, the more likely it is that the student is not in their least restrictive environment for receiving a Free and Appropriate Public Education. Unfortunately, interpreters are often placed with students who are not ready for interpreter services in lieu of providing the student direct instruction from a qualified TOD. While educational interpreters do spend time doing direct instruction, it is not what interpreters are trained for and therefore not an appropriate way for them to spend most of their time. Therefore, if you are doing direct instruction much of the time to fill in gaps in student knowledge, you will want to track the amount of time you spend doing direct instruction versus interpreting and bring that to the Individualized Education Program (IEP) Team to discuss other services the student may need.

When you are in a general education classroom with a student who is not receiving a great deal of SPED services, you may spend much more time interpreting than doing any other responsibilities. When working with a younger student, expect to spend more time doing direct instruction than when working with older students. Younger students are still learning how to use an interpreter, still acquiring their language, and still acquiring an understanding of the world to be able to map academic concepts onto background knowledge. When you work in a classroom with younger students, you may also be a helpful employee by doing such things as assisting students with tying their shoes or zipping up jackets before going outside for recess.

While you are working in a resource room, you may be doing more team liaising between the SPED teacher, the TOD, the general education teacher, and other service providers, as well as interpreting for *specially designed instruction* the Deaf student is receiving from the SPED teacher.

If you are working in a self-contained classroom, you will likely do much more of direct instruction, helpful employee, and advocating tasks than you might expect. Students in self-contained classrooms, or even resource classrooms for much of their school day, typically have a paraprofessional who does a lot of reviewing and reteaching with them—this is true of hearing students, but not always of Deaf students. Often, the interpreter is tasked with performing both interpreter and paraeducator duties for Deaf students. It is appropriate for an interpreter to do some review and reteaching, but if that is how they are spending the bulk of their time, their role is no longer that of an educational interpreter but more of a paraeducator. In such cases, the IEP Team should discuss the student's needs and then determine what type or types of service providers the student needs.

If you are working at a school for the Deaf, your role may look quite different. You may interpret for students when they take classes at a local public school in a general education mainstream setting. You may interpret classes from ASL into English for students who are using primarily spoken English and beginning to learn ASL. You will likely also interpret many more staff meetings than you would if you were an educational interpreter in a regular public school, in which case you function as both an interpreter for Deaf students and an interpreter for Deaf adults.

If you find yourself in a placement where your responsibilities are consistently something other than interpreting, it is a good idea to share how much time of the day you are spending performing various responsibilities. This may inform staffing decisions for the IEP Team. Since SPED services are associated with a specific amount of time (usually in minutes) based on assessed educational need, documenting the number of minutes you are spending performing each responsibility in the PIE Metaphor can assist you in talking to the educational team about the student's educational needs.

Supervision

Research indicates that the majority of educational interpreters are not supervised by interpreters. Most of the time, interpreter supervisors are not fluent in ASL and therefore cannot provide constructive feedback on these interpreting skills. Therefore, most educational interpreters are evaluated on soft skills such as teamwork, attendance, and attire. This is one of the reasons professional development is so important for educational interpreters. If you are working on your own all day every day with nobody to give you support and feedback on your skills, with Deaf students who are still acquiring their language and learning how to use an interpreter, you cannot grow as a professional. Seek opportunities to receive mentoring and feedback on your work, especially as a new practitioner in the field. Educators and administrators understand the value of mentorship. Use the analogy of support for young teaching professionals to help explain to your administrators your need for support. Many states provide training for educational interpreters at low or no cost. Seek and take advantage of these opportunities to grow your skills and network.

When considering taking a position at a school, ask in the interview about your chain of command. Ask who will supervise you, how you will be evaluated, and how they will provide feedback on your interpreting skills. Educational interpreters often find themselves at the center of role confusion. Many school staff members do not know what to make of the role of an educational interpreter because they do not fit into the "teacher" or "para" boxes. Therefore, you will often find school staff confusing you for another type of staff and asking you to do things that do not align with your role or function.

If you are asked by a supervisor to perform a function that conflicts with your role, responsibilities, or ethics, consider these respectful ways to say "no":

1 Acknowledge the request: "I understand this is important, and I appreciate you trusting me with this..."
2 State your reasons briefly: "However, I am currently working on ___, and I'm concerned about..."
3 Offer a compromise or alternative: "Could we discuss prioritizing my tasks, or is there someone else who could assist with this?"
4 Remain solution-focused: "I'd be happy to help after..."

This approach shows respect for your supervisor's authority while maintaining your boundaries and offering alternatives to still contribute.

Remember that Deaf Ed is dominated by two opposing philosophies, and those philosophies have direct implications for how you do your work as an interpreter. You will find yourself at philosophical odds with TODs, SLPs, and audiologists at times in your career. If these professionals are not in your chain of command, their opinions about your work are not orders. However, it is not collegial to blow off or put down the suggestions of colleagues. There is value in discussing how each of you approaches your work and why you make the decisions you do. This text provides a solid foundation for you to understand the educational system and your role within it, which will help you to talk to other educators.

DC: An interpreter I mentored was told by the Deaf student's TOD not to model multiple signs for a single English word because that would "confuse [the student]." The interpreter knew that advice did not make sense because some English words have multiple meanings that are signed different ways, and the student was even using those signs on their own independently, which showed that they knew those signs already. This type of situation is all too common, where teachers tell interpreters what to do or not to do. I always tell my interpreting students or apprentices that they would not tell the teacher how to teach, so why are they letting a teacher tell them how to interpret? Everyone will have their own opinions, and that is all well and good, but just because they express an opinion does not mean you have to follow it.

Working Environment

As an educational interpreter, regardless of how you are hired, you are an adult working on a campus with minors. Safety is the top priority of any school. As an adult in the educational environment, you are responsible for supporting the school in keeping all students safe. This means that safety responsibilities may sometimes override your interpreting responsibilities. Naturally, the safety of the Deaf student is your top priority. In emergency situations, Deaf students may not have access to instructions from teachers and other personnel. School systems are not built for Deaf students: alert systems are often more accessible auditorily than they are visually, information on the type of emergency is rarely visually accessible, and in lockdown situations the classroom may be pitch black.

The time for emergency training is not in the middle of an emergency. Every school will have an Emergency Operations Plan (EOP). As the person responsible for access for the Deaf student, it is your responsibility to know the school's EOP. Ensure that you have the opportunity to attend any training that the school provides on safety measures such as active shooter training, natural disaster training, and any other safety training. You will want to ensure that you understand the role and function of staff members in any safety situation so you can communicate appropriately with the student. Find out who is on the school's safety committee and talk to them about how staff can be trained in some basic emergency signs. Then, teach the student those signs, the appropriate responses when they see a staff member sign to them about an emergency, and use those signs during drills so the student has a chance to practice. Even when you are on breaks, you should know where the student is at all times and get to them in an emergency if possible.

Scheduling

In an ideal world, educational interpreters will not work with the same student for more than two or three years. For children to develop language proficiency, they need to have exposure to multiple models or users of a language. Often, for a Deaf child, the educational interpreter is the only ASL-fluent adult they have in their lives on a daily basis. Therefore, if they have only one educational interpreter for years on end, that substantially increases the risk that they are only exposed to one model or user of the language. There is also research to indicate the importance of exposure to native signers in supporting the development of metalinguistic awareness (Caselli, Hall, & Henner, 2020; Humphries et al., 2012; Morford & Mayberry, 2000). Metalinguistic awareness is the ability to use your language to talk about your language (Gombert, 1992). If you can talk about characteristics like rhyme, rhythm, alliteration, and connotation of words then you have metalinguistic skills. This is where *Deaf interpreters* and *language coaches* come in. It is important for a Deaf child to have native sign input in order to be able to develop the skill to use ASL to talk about other languages (i.e., English). Although there is undoubtedly a benefit to having the same educational interpreter throughout an academic year to build shared understanding, having the same interpreter multiple years in a row reduces the child's access to other signers and variations of the language.

It can be detrimental to the child's pragmatic development to have the same interpreter for multiple years in a row, especially for students who are already suffering from language deprivation. As an interpreter works with a student, they learn more about the student's personality, interests, and experiences. Knowledge of these things makes it easier to interpret for the student's expressive language. However, this knowledge will sometimes mask incomplete expressive language coming from the Deaf student.

DC: I was interpreting for a middle school student. The teacher asked the students to write about where they would go if they had a school bus, could put anybody they wanted on it, and could go anywhere in that bus that they wanted to go. I interpreted the prompt to the student and their response was "blue hat." This was during summer school, and I had very little prior experience with this student. Therefore, I had no idea what "blue hat" meant.

It took me, the teacher, and a paraeducator in conversation with the student for over 30 minutes to figure out that the location they were referring to is the NASCAR races in Florida. In the movie Cars, *there are mechanics that work on the vehicles at the races. These mechanics wear blue hats. This is the connection that the student was making. If I had some history with this student, and understood how much they love the movie* Cars, *I probably would have seen this come up in conversation before and understood they meant the NASCAR races. However, interpreting it as such based on "blue hat" would have masked the fact that the student did not communicate clearly, with context needed for communication partners, where they wanted to go. This would have masked the student's underdeveloped pragmatic skills as well as their lack of Theory of Mind.*

An additional consideration for having one interpreter with the same student for a period of time is exposure to primarily non-native ASL. Most interpreters are not native language users of ASL and therefore are not modeling native language to the Deaf student. It can be detrimental for the student to develop their language exclusively through a single second language user of ASL. If you work in a school district where you are the only interpreter, especially if you are in a rural area, this issue becomes quite sticky. You may be the only interpreter in the student's town, and therefore there may not be opportunities for them to have different educational interpreters. The student may also not have access to a larger Deaf community. This is an issue that you should bring up with the IEP Team explicitly, as the student needs to be exposed to other language models.

In such cases, it would be beneficial to build in opportunities for the student to see other language models via online means. This could include videos, translated books with native signer models, connections with other school districts in the state to provide virtual social opportunities for Deaf students, requesting an interpreting agency to send an interpreter periodically to the school in order to expose the student to other interpreting styles, finding information about community events in nearby towns to give to the teacher to share with the parents, contacting the school for the Deaf to see what kind of support or services they may have for social opportunities for the student with other signers, and offering to mentor new graduates from interpreter programs in order to bring more interpreters to your area. If you work in a school district where there are multiple interpreters, either employed by the district or employed in different buildings, it would be beneficial to work with your administration to rotate the interpreting assignments every couple of years.

Professional Development

Educational interpreters should develop an annual *Professional Development Plan* (PDP) and actively seek out professional development that addresses their professional growth. A thorough review of an educational interpreter's EIPA results is helpful in identifying skills that should be incorporated into the PDP.

While attending school district in-service training on Professional Development (PD) days has value, generally those trainings are for all district employees and not specifically for interpreters. Instead, PD days should accommodate an educational interpreter's need to attend professional development opportunities specifically designed for educational interpreters. Many educational interpreters prefer to not work on PD days and use some system of *flexible time* to attend a weekend training for educational interpreters. School districts should provide some financial assistance to pursue such opportunities; however, the availability of these resources may vary depending on the system. Many states have summer conferences for educational interpreters at little to no cost, and NAIE has a national conference every two years. Such events are vital for educational interpreters, who often work in isolation, as they provide opportunities for training, networking, and sharing effective practices.

In the Classroom

As discussed in chapter seven, the educational interpreter's role has multiple responsibilities that go above and beyond interpreting between two languages. This section delves into issues that arise in educational settings where interpreters need to have clear professional and ethical boundaries. These boundaries will likely not be understood by the educational team, so it will be the interpreter's responsibility to engage in professional discussions with their colleagues about these issues. Where appropriate, we have included suggestions for how interpreters can offer support to the Deaf student and the educational team while remaining within the boundaries of the scope of their professional practice.

Classroom Logistics

Deaf students cannot look at one thing while also "listening" to the teacher since they have to split their attention between the teacher and the interpreter. This is why Deaf teachers allow students time to look at a visual before proceeding with instruction. As an educational interpreter, you need to remember Deaf student visual needs as you position yourself in the classroom. Try to stand near any visual materials that the student may need to reference during a teacher's lesson. If you are interpreting for a student who is relying heavily on listening to the teacher using their Hearing Assistive Technology (HAT) system, consider placing yourself near the teacher, even if this means following them around the room. This will provide the student with both visual and auditory stimulus in the same locus, which will make it easier for them to look at you, the teacher, and the visuals. Sometimes, you will need to sit close to the student, and other times it may be more appropriate for you to stand farther away.

For younger students, you will likely need to position yourself closer to the student in order to assist them in directing their attention to the appropriate places in the room. As they mature, your position in the classroom will become more distant from them and closer to the teacher. Always keep the student's visual field at the top of your mind when determining where to place yourself in a classroom. Also, remember that students, especially elementary-aged students, are still learning how to use interpreters and they may not know that they have options about where to have you sit or stand. They may not know that they are missing information when they are not looking at you. If they are unsure what works for them, model different options and encourage them to select the placement where they are most comfortable having you stand. If the student is having difficulty expressing what they think is best, or does not seem to have an opinion, watch how they are paying attention in class and determine what seems to work for them regarding where you position yourself. Paying attention to where they are looking and how well they seem to have access to the classroom can give you clues into the best placement for you.

Downtime

While you will work by yourself most of the time in an educational setting, and therefore may not have many breaks, there will be times when you have downtime in the classroom. This may be while students are playing games during gym, while students are doing independent work, or while students are working with another related service provider. During these times, take advantage of the opportunity to review materials, to pull up additional visuals that you may need to support the student's language access, to talk with the teacher about their goals for upcoming lessons, or to do other related prep. Do not look at downtime as "free time," but as time to leverage to prepare for working with the student. Often, educational interpreters do not receive paid prep time. However, downtime during classes can be converted into paid prep time by using that time wisely. If the teachers understand that you are engaged in an activity that is going to further the support you provide for the Deaf student, they are less likely to interrupt that time to ask you to perform other tasks.

Behavior Management

One of the most common concerns of working educational interpreters is how to handle requests for behavior management. The phrase "behavior is communication" particularly applies to Deaf children with language deprivation. Certain behaviors are common for children with language deprivation. These include eloping (leaving the classroom without permission), refusing to look at the interpreter or the teacher, hitting, kicking, biting, and throwing things. In educational settings, when a child's behavior is considered atypical for their age, there may be a *Behavior Intervention Plan* (BIP) in place. In order to have a BIP, the student must first have a functional behavioral assessment (FBA) that documents how they behave in different environments. The BIP is a part of the IEP. If an interpreter is working with a student who has a BIP, it is important for them to know their specific responsibilities regarding this plan. They also need to know what is included in the BIP so they can provide appropriate, consistent support to the student.

However, behavior management is not the sole responsibility of an educational interpreter. A student with significant behavioral concerns in the classroom requires further support, such as that of a paraeducator. In a perfect world, a Deaf child on an IEP with a BIP would have both an educational interpreter and a paraeducator. However, as this is not a perfect world, interpreters are often seen as responsible for managing student behavior. Interpreters must be able to appropriately explain to administration that it is impossible to engage in actions, such as *Crisis Prevention Intervention* (CPI) holds, and also interpret at the same time (Crisis Prevention Institute, 2020). If a child is experiencing emotional dysregulation, and having significant behaviors, the interpreter will need the support of other staff members so they can interpret during these times. You cannot perform a CPI hold and also interpret. Furthermore, the use of CPI holds requires specific initial training and annual refresher training.

In situations where a student's safety is at risk, the educational interpreter is to act as a staff member according to the school handbook to ensure safety for everyone involved. This may require them to stop interpreting briefly in order to address a safety concern.

Social Interaction

Ask any student what they like best about school and most of the time their answer will include something about hanging out with friends. Social interaction is a critical part of the educational experience for all students, and it is an area where educational interpreters have to exercise sound judgment. In early elementary grades, students will see you as another adult in the environment and will not necessarily think very much of your role in interpreting interactions between them and their peers.

However, as students enter middle school, social interaction and peer groups become a defining characteristic of their lives. This is an area where you as an interpreter will see the greatest impact of your gender, race, age, and lived experience (i.e., most interpreters are white women, but the majority of Deaf students are not). One of the defining characteristics of teenage communication is selective sharing. As children go through puberty, they start to develop a sense of privacy, and they stop sharing openly with everyone and begin to be more selective about what they say, and to whom. This type of differentiation is a natural part of pragmatic development. This means that students will start to see their educational interpreter's presence as more intrusive in certain conversations. Therefore, be aware of how you are being perceived by the student and their peers, and how the Deaf student is being perceived through you as you interpret social interactions.

It may be beneficial for you to provide additional support as needed for the student to be able to communicate independently with their peers through texting, writing notes, gesturing, or using some ASL. You may also need to have a direct conversation with the student's peers so they understand that everything you interpret is kept confidential, except in the cases of things that must be reported by law or by school policy. Your responsibility as an educational interpreter is to support the student's autonomy. During opportunities for social interaction, make yourself available, but do not impose on the student as they get older.

Teaching ASL

In the Deaf community, the role of ASL teacher is exclusively for Deaf people. Therefore, it is inappropriate for hearing educational interpreters to teach ASL. That said, there may be times in which hearing students want to learn some social phrases or some signs to be able to communicate with their Deaf peers. For younger students, the interpreter may provide more direct support in this area, but for older students, interpreters should encourage Deaf students to model the signs for their peers as they are interested in learning. In secondary settings, it is common for students to have clubs around a variety of topics.

If the school wants to have an ASL club, the educational interpreter should be there to support Deaf students in sharing their language, not as an ASL teacher. Interpreters should be prepared to share resources for where individuals may go and learn ASL from Deaf sources. Share resources that are available via popular social media apps, as these are what hearing students are more likely to use.

Ironically, as an educational interpreter, you may end up in the position of teaching ASL to the Deaf student. According to the NAIE's national survey, about 50% of Deaf students did not know any ASL before being assigned an educational interpreter. Therefore, your responsibilities may be less about teaching ASL to hearing peers and staff, and more about supporting the ASL development of the student with whom you are working. This is a sticky situation to be in. A student cannot learn their foundational language when they are learning content through an interpretation (Caselli, Hall, & Henner, 2020; Monikowski, 2004; Peterson & Monikowski, 2010). Therefore, if you are working with a student who does not have fluency in ASL, you should be aware of resources you can use to expose them to native language models. While it may not be possible to have a native language model in school (i.e., *Deaf interpreter* or *language coach*, for which you absolutely should advocate), there are video resources online that you can use to support the student's language development in that way.

Testing Considerations

In chapter four, we covered testing and high-stakes testing. However, this topic bears mentioning again as it is *critical* for educational interpreters to understand the goal and function of any kind of test before deciding how, or if, to interpret it. In general, any support or accommodations for testing should be outlined in the student's IEP. Therefore, this is the first place where an interpreter should look before making decisions about interpreting tests. As a general rule of thumb, it is a good idea not to interpret any passages on a test that have been included to evaluate reading comprehension.

A common conundrum for educational interpreters is spelling tests, and how to handle interpreting word lists when there are no ASL equivalents. Spelling tests are common and cannot be proctored in print, so most educational interpreters must interpret them in their careers. There are different perspectives on how to handle such tests. Some people will tell you to fingerspell on a spelling test based on research with native signers that shows they do not process every letter in a fingerspelled word to access meaning (Emmorey & Corina, 1990; Wilcox, 1992). Others will make up a sign for the moment that you only use for that test (Schick, Williams, & Kupermintz, 2006). This is not good advice. Others will say to use cues such as Visual Phonics (Kart, 2021; Narr, 2008; Trezek & Malmgren, 2005), which should be done only if the student already uses such a system *and* if you have been trained in that system. In reality, there is no perfect answer to this question.

We believe lexicalized-like fingerspelling is the best approach for interpreting spelling tests for words that do not have a sign equivalent (Alawad & Musyoka, 2018; Fitzmaurice, 2024; Haptonstall-Nykaza & Shick, 2007; Roos, 2013; Stone, Kartheiser, Hauser, Petitto, & Allen, 2015). In *lexicalized fingerspelling*, only the first and last letters of the word are discernible (Valli, Lucas, Mulrooney, & Villanueva, 2011). In ASL, lexicalized fingerspelling consists of signs that began as fingerspelled words and, over time, have taken on a set meaning and the properties of proper ASL signs—they have a path movement, a beginning and ending handshape, and a fixed meaning. By using this natural process to create lexicalized-like fingerspelled words during a spelling test, interpreters are giving information that is visually equivalent to the auditory information a teacher gives hearing students.

When teachers dictate words for a spelling test, they often emphasize the sounds in the words. They do this to clue students into possible spelling patterns based on how the word sounds. Whereas fingerspelling didactically, or letter by letter, would give too much information, lexicalized-like fingerspelling gives similar visual cues to the information hearing children can glean from the teacher's auditory cues. Spelling tests are always based on lists of words that the student has seen before. Therefore, they should need little prompting to identify which word they are supposed to write come test time. If any word must be presented with lexicalized-like fingerspelling, the interpreter should model what this looks like for each word before the spelling test.

Preparation

Many educational interpreters believe that effective preparation of materials only requires pre-reading the content and/or looking at the teacher's PowerPoint materials. Evidence indicates this is absolutely not an effective preparation technique. Preparation is best rooted in understanding teacher discourse. This allows educational interpreters to move away from word-for-word interpreting attempts and to move toward taking advantage of classroom discourse to shape interpreting decisions.

Again, word-for-sign strategies are rooted in *conduit models* of interpreting and are highly ineffective in educational settings. Teacher discourse is aimed at promoting higher-order thinking, social engagement, and scaffolded content and interactions. A discourse lens helps students learn by providing keywords and phrases from which to process information. This means understanding how teachers talk is key to good preparation.

Passive preparation types such as pre-reading or pre-viewing textbooks and PowerPoint materials *may* be helpful in terms of making educational interpreters feel more confident in their individual understanding of the material. However, after extensive analyses, there is no actual significant benefit to such passive preparation approaches. It does not actually make a better interpretation.

What is needed to actually prepare is to review the instructional curriculum guides for each subject at that grade level and put your hands up and practice interpreting the key vocabulary. This type of preparation creates more pathways to your memory, so the material is more readily accessible when you actually interpret (Nicodemus, Swabey, & Taylor, 2014; Russell & Winston, 2014; Russell, Williamson, Hayes, & Nelson-Julander, 2021).

It is also key for educational interpreters to be aware of teacher discourse. Teachers use a variety of discourse styles to manage their classrooms and student learning (Cazden, 2001). These include soliciting student participation (as previously discussed with the initiate, respond, and evaluate (IRE) structure), orienting (providing directions), semantic organizational cues (contextual and incidental language learning), developing metacognitive (higher-order) thinking, and, of course, providing main ideas (found in the curricula). Some of these discourse strategies can be directly found in the revised *Bloom's Taxonomy* (Anderson & Krathwohl, 2001; Bloom, 1956), sometimes referred to as Depth of Knowledge (DOK) levels.

SF: It is interesting that on the occasion I am teaching a class in English, hearing students are all adept at knowing when to perk up and what information is important just by monitoring my speech pattern. They all know (just as many of you do) when to perk up and listen for "what is on the test" etc. As educational interpreters, we have to listen for those discourse cues as well and ensure we interpret that discursive shift effectively—what follows should never be omitted.

DC: Furthermore, Deaf students cannot passively scan for these shifts visually the way that hearing people can scan for them auditorily. It may be appropriate to use a visual attention-getting strategy to provide the Deaf student with an opportunity to choose to cue into the information.

Ideally, educational interpreters have preparation time built into their schedules as well as office space.

SF: I have heard many educational interpreters share that they do not have preparation time in their schedule. However, when you identify they are compensated for 7.5 hours a day and are only interpreting for 6.5 hours a day—it means the preparation time is built into their schedule as a before or after school hours activity. I also hear many educational interpreters lamenting the fact they do not have office space for preparation. We all know office space is a rare and valuable commodity in overcrowded schools. For me, I would rather prepare at home where it is quiet anyway—well, at least quieter than at a school.

To make effective use of preparation time, for obvious reasons, educational interpreters must have access to copies of texts, scripts, notes, and videos. Educational interpreters also need time for preparation as well as time to consult with teachers to figure out what is coming up in the classroom.

While many educational interpreters want teacher daily lesson plans, in reality, that is not likely a battle worth fighting. Frankly, it is easier for an educational interpreter to ask for tomorrow's PowerPoint presentation and what they hope students will "take away from tomorrow's lesson" in the few minutes transitioning to a new period or lesson. This helps with pre-teaching too.

Pre-Teaching (AKA Tutoring)

Unfortunately, the model of mainstream education seems stuck in the notion of providing tutoring or providing an intervention after the material has been taught. Although tutoring is an effective strategy for students who need extra practice or additional time, it is always essentially a catch-up game.

We strongly advocate replacing tutoring with pre-teaching material (Antia, Jones, Reed, & Kreimeyer, 2009; Fitzmaurice, 2021a; 2021b; Luckner & Cooke, 2010; Marschark, Lang, & Albertini, 2002; Schick, Williams, & Kupermintz, 2006). Pre-teaching is a highly effective instructional strategy to help Deaf students understand key vocabulary and general concepts before attending the class lesson.

SF: It makes far more sense to pre-teach the key vocabulary and foundational knowledge beforehand. That way, when the Deaf student is in the class, they can find benefit in the classroom instruction, whereas tutoring means the Deaf student does not understand the material in the lesson and has to wait for it to make sense later in a tutoring session. That seems like a huge waste of precious time.

In terms of pre-teaching vocabulary, first and foremost, you will need to identify vocabulary and key terms. These can be found by checking the state curriculum, textbooks, and having brief conversations with teachers. If you remember interpreting for academic subjects from chapter four, we discussed the *sandwich technique* and helping students decode printed text (Fitzmaurice, 2024). Pre-teaching key vocabulary using the *sandwich technique* is vital. For example: T-R-E-E (fingerspelled) + TREE (sign) + T-R-E-E (fingerspelled). The *sandwich* approach provides the Deaf student the opportunity to link the fingerspelling to the sign.

Again, just as English creates compound words (e.g., notebook, blueberry, blackboard), ASL is a heavily compounding language (Klima & Bellugi, 1979; Liddell & Johnson, 1986). Ultimately, compounding often creates a new word or sign which is different from the component parts of that word or sign. This is important because, oftentimes, there are no commonly used ASL signs for much of English's lexicon.

For example, if an educational interpreter notices *habitat* as part of the key vocabulary, they will need to create a compound to represent that concept. It could look like: NATURAL HOME ANIMAL PLANT. Again, the compound represents the concept and becomes the de facto, interim sign for habitat. Using the *sandwich technique*, the key vocabulary looks like: H-A-B-I-T-A-T NATURAL HOME ANIMAL PLANT H-A-B-I-T-A-T. This should be followed up with visuals, pictures, or videos. And, as with any concept, repetition is important for student retention.

Pre-teaching vocabulary in this proactive way provides Deaf students with foundational knowledge *before* they enter the class lesson and supports their learning *during* the lesson. As a side benefit, it reduces anxiety among Deaf students and increases classroom participation because the students will be better prepared.

Your Health and Well-Being

As an educational interpreter, you will likely work alone during the school day without the support of a team interpreter. While there are frequent breaks in academic instruction, there will be situations in which you may have to interpret for a long stretch of time without a break.

The most common physical injury that interpreters experience is repetitive motion injury. Canadian researchers found 25% of interpreters have been diagnosed with a repetitive injury such as tendonitis or carpal tunnel syndrome (Fischer, Marshall, & Woodcock, 2012). Interpreters reported the greatest discomfort is in the neck, right forearm (for right-handed signers), hand, and wrist.

Tendonitis is inflammation of the tendons between your muscles and bones causing pain at the tendon site and surrounding area. Carpal tunnel syndrome is where the nerves that run down the arm, through the wrist, and into the fingers become pinched over time, leading to numbness in the fingers.

It is critical for educational interpreters to have good posture, ergonomic seating, and built-in breaks (Fischer & Woodcock, 2012; Johnson & Feuerstein, 2005).

Stretching, massage therapy, heat (warm up beforehand) or ice treatments (cool down afterwards), and strengthening exercises for your shoulders, back, arms, and wrists will all reduce the likelihood of repetitive motion injuries.

Educational interpreters should also take as many micro-breaks from interpreting as possible, which look like behind-the-back stretches and wrist rotations. If an educational interpreter feels the need to wear a brace (while not interpreting) to help an injury heal, that can be beneficial. Again, though, do not interpret in a brace designed to immobilize your forearm—this leads to further injury. If you are so sore you need to keep the brace on, inquire about medical leave.

Working in educational settings, there are other risks for physical injury. Aside from the stress on the body of interpreting for long periods of time, another potential source of physical injury is from student behavior. If a student has a violent dysregulation, you might be injured. You might be interpreting a physical education class or after-school sport and be hit by a rogue ball. Any time you experience a physical injury at work, follow the protocols that your school has set out for employees when they experience workplace injuries.

You may also be exposed to bloodborne pathogens. Your school will have training and procedures in place addressing what you should do in the event of an exposure. If you are an agency-placed interpreter, ask the school's front desk for a copy of their procedures around bloodborne pathogens.

Emotional Trauma

Educational interpreting can be emotionally exhausting for several interconnected reasons. At the heart of the interpreter's role is a commitment to equity, access, and inclusion—yet interpreters are often placed in systems that were not built with Deaf students in mind. This systemic mismatch creates an ongoing tension that interpreters must navigate daily.

You will be working alongside a Deaf student in a school system overwhelmingly designed for hearing children, where spoken language and auditory learning are assumed to be the norm. Many classrooms rely heavily on verbal explanations, group discussions, incidental learning, and auditory cues—things Deaf students may miss even with an interpreter present. As the interpreter, you often witness these gaps and experience the emotional strain of seeing the student left out, even when you are doing your best to provide access.

You will likely encounter professionals who frame deafness as a deficit, viewing it primarily as a medical condition to be fixed rather than as a cultural and linguistic identity. This deficit mindset can lead to decisions that devalue ASL, overlook Deaf cultural norms, and push technologies like cochlear implants without considering the full linguistic and social needs of the student. Being part of meetings or classrooms where the student's identity is misunderstood or minimized can be disheartening and ethically challenging for interpreters.

Additionally, you may work with teachers who are unfamiliar with how Deaf students learn best, especially if they lack training in visual learning strategies or Deaf education. Teachers may not modify their instruction for visual accessibility, may speak too fast, use idioms, or fail to engage directly with the Deaf student. The interpreter often bears the burden of bridging these gaps while simultaneously maintaining professional impartiality—a balance that can feel impossible when a student's needs are not being met.

Over time, this emotional labor—the constant vigilance, advocacy, and silent witnessing of inequities—can lead to compassion fatigue or burnout. Interpreters care deeply about Deaf students and often feel powerless within the larger system. Without proper support, collaboration, and acknowledgment of these systemic challenges, the role can become isolating, ethically ambiguous, and emotionally draining.

In your career, you may be the only person with whom the Deaf student can communicate—at school or at home. You will face the challenging task of giving a Deaf student language and access to academic material at the same time. You will witness the effects of language deprivation, information deprivation, and other forms of trauma that Deaf children experience. You will personally witness the struggles that a Deaf student has with their educational experiences and will frequently feel like you are screaming into the void when you try to do something about it. Often, you will do this alone. It is important as an educational interpreter that you have a support system to address what you experience during your career. Unaddressed emotional trauma leads to burnout and can have lasting effects on you and the Deaf students you serve.

DC: I once interpreted for a student who spent every school break in a movie theater. When they returned to school after break, they would be bursting with questions about the movies they watched because they had nobody who could communicate with them at home.

Burnout

Burnout is a response to chronic work demands involving significant interpersonal obligations, with emotional exhaustion being a key component (Bower, 2015; Humphrey, 2015; Massengale, 2024; Schwenke, 2015; Swartz, 2008). Though precise burnout rates for interpreters, especially educational interpreters, are not well-documented, high turnover and reports of burnout suggest it is a significant issue.

Causes of Burnout

There are several causes of burnout including cumulative trauma or frequent exposure to distressing situations. Role overload, role ambiguity, and unrealistic expectations are other causes of burnout for educational interpreters (Fitzmaurice, 2021b).

An additional cause of burnout is high stress levels from managing demanding responsibilities—certainly a hallmark of educational interpreting. High stress levels, and the associated response, can have physiological effects such as increased levels of stress hormones like cortisol, which can degrade interpretation quality. High stress levels can lead to emotional and physical exhaustion.

Another factor particular to interpreters is the perception of a lack of control. Interpreters who feel they have more control over their work experience lower levels of burnout compared to those who feel less control. We highly recommend using the Demand-Control Schema (Dean & Pollard, 2001; 2013) in light of Role Space as these frameworks help educational interpreters to maximize the decision latitude they have, which increases the perception of control.

Witnessing continuous oppression can also be a cause of burnout. Observing power imbalances, audism, racism, and feeling part of the oppressive group(s) can lead to guilt and self-victimization, affecting self-care.

Symptoms of Burnout

Burnout is often evident through emotional exhaustion such as ongoing fatigue, strain, frustration, and a general sense of feeling drained. Interpreters may also begin to experience depersonalization, disconnection from the work, and a lower sense of personal accomplishment (Maslach, Schaufeli, & Leiter, 2001; Pines & Aronson, 1988). As a result, interpreters may distance themselves from their work.

Other symptoms of burnout include persistent feelings of inadequacy and frustration with work or with interactions with others. This comes with feelings of helplessness and the belief that nothing will improve or feeling overwhelmed by the demands of the job. This is often accompanied by an overwhelming sense of self-doubt about job performance and general negative or cynical feelings. These feelings are compounded by a lack of oversight from supervisors who are knowledgeable in the field of interpreting or capable of providing meaningful feedback about interpreting work.

These emotions can manifest themselves into physical symptoms such as:

- Chronic Fatigue: Persistent tiredness not alleviated by rest.
- Sleep Disturbances: Difficulty falling asleep, staying asleep, or experiencing unrestful sleep.
- Headaches and Muscle Tension: Frequent headaches or muscle pain, especially in the neck and shoulders.
- Gastrointestinal Issues: Stomach problems, such as nausea or indigestion.
- Concentration Problems: Difficulty focusing or maintaining attention.
- Memory Issues: Trouble remembering details or important information.
- Decision-Making Difficulties: Struggling with making decisions or solving problems effectively.
- Emotional Numbness: Feeling emotionally flat or detached from work or personal life.

The above physical symptoms can then change an interpreter's behavior to include:

- Withdrawal: Increasing isolation from colleagues or social activities.
- Decreased Performance: A noticeable drop in work productivity and quality.
- Procrastination: Avoiding tasks and putting off responsibilities.
- Increased Absenteeism: Frequent absences from work or increased use of sick leave.

Strategies to Avoid Burnout

The first strategy includes self-awareness. If you recognize and understand your personal stressors and the stressful job demands of educational interpreting, you can avoid burnout altogether.

Interpreting for students subjected to high-stakes testing and routine examination of their comprehension of the curricular materials which they access through your interpreting work, often with language deprivation, are stressful! Aside from burnout, lack of stress management can become a significant health concern.

Develop coping strategies and self-care routines. Self-care means taking care of your body, mind, spirit, and relationships. For interpreters from traditionally minoritized groups, factors affecting burnout are multiplied by living in oppressive systems. We recognize that self-care is often a privilege not afforded to all. Sometimes life demands more than we have the space, time, and resources to give. To the extent possible, try to incorporate some of these standard prescriptions we usually forget, particularly in times of high stress:

- Eat healthy
- Drink plenty of water
- Exercise (work out, walk, yoga, dance)
- Sleep
- Floss
- Read books for fun
- Create something (bake, do art, write, play music, sew, crochet, color, build Lego)
- Meditate or pray
- Do random acts of kindness
- Spend time with family and friends

Develop healthy habits and routines so they are easier to do and maintain. This will ultimately help educational interpreters sustain performance and avoid burnout in many aspects of life.

DC: I do all the things. ALL the things. I have had to learn over time how to have balance. It began when I was a grad student, and my husband started buying me a book to read for fun when I was flying somewhere for a research trip or conference. He wanted me to read on the plane instead of working because I worked ALL THE TIME. Now, I have specific times in my schedule blocked out for soul-feeding activities. I meet with my best friend on Zoom in the mornings before work. I book a monthly massage. I attend church with my family. I have weekly dance classes. I make coffee dates with my son. I leave at least one night a week free to only spend with my family, and at least one weekend a month. We do grocery shopping together once a week. I go to bed early so I can read a book for pleasure before I go to sleep. I sleep seven to nine hours a night. Whenever humanly possible, I do not let work interfere with these times.

In addition, educational interpreters should develop a network of confidants to debrief with. Dean and Pollard (2001) note, "traditionally, interpreters have been taught that thoughts, information, commentary and feelings are to be suppressed..." (p. 6). This is false. Find confidants to debrief with regularly (Fitzmaurice & Faulkner, 2023). Make it a weekly habit! The professional term for this is *case conferencing*. It is vital to effective reflective practice.

We are both big advocates of counseling. Despite the social stigma, seek counseling services, which are often available at little cost through Employee Assistance Programs (EAPs). We both do.

Managing stress by enacting meaningful routines will stop much of the burnout triggers for educational interpreters. Do not abandon those when stress levels increase significantly. Use the Demand-Control Schema, find a confidant, and use counseling services as needed. Use the word "no." Sometimes you just have to admit you cannot do it all and selectively take things off of your plate. Do so. We cannot afford to lose you to burnout.

Summary

Educational interpreting is a profession that demands both strong cognitive abilities and key personality traits. This chapter discussed that interpreters must quickly process complex linguistic information, often in fast-paced classroom environments, while managing emotional challenges such as witnessing oppression or working with minimal support. Cognitive skills like rapid reasoning, working memory, and task switching are essential, especially when interpreting for Deaf students who may have limited language development. Personality traits such as emotional stability, empathy, patience, and flexibility play a crucial role in managing stress, fostering teamwork, and making ethical decisions.

The EIPA evaluates interpreters across multiple domains but serves as a diagnostic tool rather than formal certification. Although many states use the EIPA to establish minimum standards, requirements vary widely, and no national certification currently exists. Organizations like the NAIE are actively exploring options for a unified certification to enhance professional standards and consistency.

This chapter also addressed how educational interpreters may be employed by school districts, regional education programs, or interpreting agencies. Understanding the student's language needs, expected duties, and working conditions is critical before accepting a position. Interpreter roles vary depending on placement, with responsibilities ranging from direct interpretation to advocacy and instructional support. Excessive time spent in non-interpreting roles can signal inadequate service provision and raise concerns about meeting students' educational rights.

Many interpreters work without direct supervision from ASL-fluent professionals, often receiving evaluations based on attendance or teamwork rather than interpreting skills. Mentoring and constructive feedback are vital for professional growth. Interpreters should seek clarity on evaluation processes and advocate for support systems similar to those provided for educators. Ongoing professional development tailored to interpreting, rather than general district training, is key to maintaining and advancing skills.

Beyond interpreting, educational interpreters must navigate complex classroom logistics and maintain clear professional boundaries. Positioning is important to ensure Deaf students have visual access to the interpreter, teacher, and materials. Interpreters must balance social interaction, respect student privacy, and avoid assuming inappropriate roles such as teaching ASL or managing behavior. Ethical challenges often arise from role confusion and differing philosophies within Deaf education, requiring tactful communication and collaboration with educational teams.

Effective preparation involves more than reviewing content; interpreters must understand teaching styles, discourse patterns, and curriculum goals. Access to classroom materials and collaboration with teachers support successful pre-teaching, which is more beneficial than tutoring after class. Interpreters should also be familiar with appropriate strategies for interpreting tests, including specialized techniques for spelling tests and ensuring fidelity to the test format.

Interpreters face physical risks such as repetitive strain injuries and must prioritize ergonomic practices, stretching, and injury prevention. Emotional trauma from systemic challenges, isolation, and heavy emotional labor is common, potentially leading to burnout. To sustain their health and effectiveness, interpreters should develop self-awareness, practice self-care, maintain support networks, set boundaries, and seek counseling when needed. Proactive strategies to manage workload and stress contribute to career longevity and quality interpreting services.

Thought Questions

1 What questions will you ask in the process of applying or interviewing for a job as an educational interpreter? How can these questions help you make ethically sound decisions about which educational interpreter jobs to take or turn down?
2 What is the sandwich technique? How can it be used by educational interpreters to enhance the pre-teaching of vocabulary for Deaf students?
3 In what ways does pre-teaching key vocabulary and concepts benefit Deaf students in the classroom? What impact does this teaching have on their participation and anxiety levels?
4 How do personality traits such as emotional stability, conscientiousness, and flexibility contribute to the effectiveness of an educational interpreter? Why are these traits particularly important in educational settings as opposed to other areas in which interpreters may work?
5 What are the signs of burnout in interpreting? Have you experienced any symptoms of high stress and, if so, which ones? How do you (or can you) address those symptoms? What steps can you take to prevent these symptoms from occurring in the first place?
6 What is one self-care technique that you already employ? Is it effective in relieving stress or symptoms of burnout? What other techniques can you begin to employ now?

References

Alawad, H., & Musyoka, M. (2018). Examining the effectiveness of fingerspelling in improving the vocabulary and literacy skills of deaf students. *Creative Education*, 9 (3), 456–468.

Anderson, L. W., & Krathwohl, D. R. (Eds.). (2001). *A taxonomy for learning, teaching, and assessing: A revision of Bloom's taxonomy of educational objectives*. New York: Longman.

Angelelli, C. V. (2004). *Medical interpreting and cross-cultural communication*. New York: Cambridge University Press.

Antia, S. D., Jones, P., Reed, S., & Kreimeyer, K. H. (2009). Academic status and progress of deaf and hard-of-hearing students in general education classrooms. *Journal of Deaf Studies and Deaf Education*, 14(3), 293–311.

ASL Interpreting. (n.d.). The RID ED:K-12 certificate moratorium. Edmonton: Interpreting Consolidated. https://www.aslinterpreting.com/the-rid-edk-12-certificate-moratorium/.

Bloom, B. S. (1956). *Taxonomy of educational objectives, handbook 1: The cognitive domain*. London: McKay Co.

Bontempo, K., & Napier, J. (2007). Mind the gap! A skills analysis of sign language interpreters. *The Sign Language Translator and Interpreter*, 1(2), 275–299.

Bower, M. (2015). *Burnout of sign language interpreters: A comparative study of K-12, post-secondary, and community interpreters* (Master's thesis). Western Oregon University.

Campbell, J. P., McCloy, R. A., Oppler, S. H., & Sager, C. E. (1993). A theory of performance. In N. Schmitt & W. C. Borman (Eds.), *Personnel selection in organizations* (pp. 35–70). San Francisco, CA: Jossey-Bass.

Caselli, N. K., Hall, W. C., & Henner, J. (2020). American Sign Language interpreters in public schools: An Illusion of inclusion that perpetuates language deprivation. *Maternal and Child Health Journal*, 24(11), 1323–1329.

Cates, D. (2021). Patterns in EIPA test scores and implications for interpreter education. *Journal of Interpretation*, 29(1), 6.

Cates, D., & Delkamiller, J. (2021). The impact of sign language interpreter skill on education outcomes in K–12 settings. In E. A. Winston & S. B. Fitzmaurice (Eds.), *Advances in educational interpreting* (pp. 19–30). Washington, DC: Gallaudet University Press.

Cazden, C. B. (2001). *Classroom discourse: The language of teaching and learning* (2nd ed.). Cambridge, MA: Harvard University Press.

Crisis Prevention Institute. (2020). *Nonviolent crisis intervention: Participant workbook* (3rd ed.). Milwaukee, WI: Crisis Prevention Institute.

Dean, R. K., & Pollard, R. Q. (2001). Application of demand-control theory to sign language interpreting: Implications for stress and interpreter training. *Journal of Deaf Studies and Deaf Education*, 6(1), 1–14.

Dean, R. K., & Pollard, R. Q. (2013). *The demand control schema: Interpreting as a practice profession*. Washington, DC: Gallaudet University Press.

Educational Interpreter Performance Assessment (EIPA). (n.d.). About the EIPA. https://www.eipaassessment.com/about-eipa.

Emmorey, K., & Corina, D. (1990). Lexical recognition in sign language: Effects of phonetic structure and morphology. *Perceptual & Motor Skills*, 71(3_suppl), 1227–1252.

Fischer, S. L., Marshall, M. M., & Woodcock, K. (2012). Musculoskeletal disorders in sign language interpreters: A systematic review and conceptual model of musculoskeletal disorder development. *WORK: A Journal of Prevention, Assessment & Rehabilitation*, 42(2), 173–184.

Fischer, S. L., & Woodcock, K. (2012). A cross-sectional survey of reported musculoskeletal pain, disorders, work volume and employment situation among sign language interpreters. *International Journal of Industrial Ergonomics*, 42(4), 335–340.

Fitzmaurice, S. (2010). Teaching goals of interpreter educators. *International Journal of Interpreter Education*, 2(1), 14–24.

Fitzmaurice, S. (2021a). The realistic role metaphor for educational interpreters. In E. A. Winston & S. B. Fitzmaurice (Eds.), *Advances in educational interpreting* (pp. 285–307). Washington, DC: Gallaudet University Press.

Fitzmaurice, S. (2021b). *The role of the educational interpreter: Perceptions of administrators and teachers*. Washington, DC: Gallaudet University Press.

Fitzmaurice, S. (2024). Importance of fingerspelling in education settings. In J. Bentley-Sassaman, R. F. Minor, & S. Fitzmaurice (Eds.), *A survey of American Sign Language/English interpreting settings* (pp. 19–32). OER Commons.

Fitzmaurice, S. B., & Faulkner, M. (2023). ASL-English interpreters and anxiety. *Journal of Interpretation*, 31(1): Article 5.

Gile, D. (2009). *Basic concepts and models for interpreter and translator training* (Rev. ed.). Amsterdam: John Benjamins.

Gile, D. (2025, March 20). The effort models and gravitational model: Clarifications and update [PowerPoint slides]. CIRIN. https://www.cirin-gile.fr/powerpoint/The-Effort-Models-and-Gravitational-Model-Clarifications-and-update.pdf.

Gombert, J. E. (1992). *Metalinguistic development*. Chicago, IL: University of Chicago Press.

Haptonstall-Nykaza, T., & Schick, B. (2007). The transition from fingerspelling to English print: Facilitating English decoding. *Journal of Deaf Studies and Deaf Education*, 12(2), 172–183.

Horváth, I. (2011). *Interpreter behaviour: A psychological approach*. Paris: L'Harmattan.

Humphrey, C. (2015). *Job satisfaction, role strain, burnout, and self-care among American Sign Language/English Interpreters* (Master's thesis). Western Oregon University.

Humphries, T., Kushalnagar, P., Mathur, G., Napoli, D. J., Padden, C., Rathmann, C., & Smith, S. R. (2012). Language acquisition for deaf children: Reducing the harms of zero tolerance to the use of alternative approaches. *Harm Reduction Journal*, 9(1): 16.

Janzen, T. (2005). Interpretation and language use: ASL and English. In T. Janzen (Ed.), *Topics in signed language interpreting: Theory and practice* (pp. 69–105). Amsterdam: John Benjamins.

Johnson, W. L., & Feuerstein, M. (2005). An interpreter's interpretation: Sign language interpreters' view of musculoskeletal disorders. *Journal of Occupational Rehabilitation*, 15(3), 401–415.

Kart, A. N. (2021). Systematic review of studies on Visual Phonics. *Communication Disorders Quarterly*, 43(4), 261–271.

Klima, E. S., & Bellugi, U. (1979). *The signs of language*. Cambridge, MA: Harvard University Press.

Liddell, S. K., & Johnson, R. E. (1986). American Sign Language compound formation processes, lexicalization, and phonological remnants. *Natural Language & Linguistic Theory*, 4(4), 445–513.

Luckner, J. L., & Cooke, C. (2010). A summary of the vocabulary research with students who are deaf or hard of hearing. *American Annals of the Deaf*, 155(1), 38–67.

Macnamara, B. N. (2009). Interpreter cognitive aptitudes. *Journal of Interpretation, 2008–2009*, 9–32.

Macnamara, B. N., Moore, A. B., Kegl, J. A., & Conway, A. R. A. (2011). Domain-general cognitive abilities and simultaneous interpreting skill. *Interpreting*, 13(1), 121–142.

Macnamara, B. N., Moore, A. B., Kegl, J. A., & Conway, A. R. A. (2014). Domain-general cognitive abilities and simultaneous interpreting skill. In F. Pöchhacker & M. Liu (Eds.), *Aptitude for interpreting* (pp. 107–128). Amsterdam: John Benjamins.

Marschark, M., Lang, H. G., & Albertini, J. A. (2002). *Educating deaf students: From research to practice*. New York: Oxford University Press.

Maslach, C., Schaufeli, W. B., & Leiter, M. P. (2001). Job burnout. *Annual Review of Psychology*, 52, 397–422.

Massengale, M. (2024, April). Preventing ASL interpreter burnout through the use of self-care. Poster presented at the Liberty University Research Symposium, Liberty University, Lynchburg, VA.

McCrae, R. R., & Costa, P. T.Jr. (1999). A five-factor theory of personality. In L. A. Pervin & O. P. John (Eds.), *Handbook of personality: Theory and research* (2nd ed., pp. 139–153). New York: Guilford Press.

Monikowski, C. (2004). Language myths in interpreted education: First language, second language, what language? In E. Winston (Ed.), *Educational interpreting: How it can succeed* (pp. 48–60). Washington, DC: Gallaudet University Press.

Morford, J. P., & Mayberry, R. I. (2000). A reexamination of "early exposure" and its implication for language acquisition by eye. In C. Chamberlain, J. P. Morford, & R. I. Mayberry (Eds.), *Language acquisition by eye* (pp. 111–127). Mahwah, NJ: Erlbaum.

Napier, J. (2004). Interpreting omissions: A new perspective. *Interpreting*, 6(2), 117–142.

Napier, J., McKee, R., & Goswell, D. (2006). *Sign language interpreting: Theory and practice in Australia and New Zealand*. Alexandria, NSW: Federation Press.

Narr, R. F. (2008). Phonological awareness and decoding in deaf/hard-of-hearing students who use Visual Phonics. *Journal of Deaf Studies and Deaf Education*, 13(3), 405–416.

National Association of Interpreters in Education (NAIE). (2023, March 31). State requirements for educational interpreters. https://naiedu.org/state-standards/.

National Association of Interpreters in Education (NAIE). (n.d.). Professional guidelines for interpreting in educational settings (1st ed.). Retrieved May 19, 2025, from https://naiedu.org/guidelines/.

National Consortium of Interpreter Education Centers (NCIEC). (2016). Educational Interpreter Performance Assessment (EIPA): Overview and score descriptions. https://www.interpretereducation.org/resources/eipa/.

Nicodemus, B., Swabey, L., & Taylor, M. (2014). Preparation strategies used by American Sign Language-English interpreters to render President Barack Obama's inaugural address. *The Interpreters Newsletter*, 19, 27–44.

Peterson, R., & Monikowski, C. (2010). Perceptions of efficacy of sign language interpreters working in K–12 settings. In K. M. Christensen (Ed.), *Ethical considerations in educating children who are deaf or hard of hearing* (pp. 129–153). Washington, DC: Gallaudet University Press.

Pines, A. M., & Aronson, E. (1988). *Career burnout: Causes and cures*. New York: Free Press.

Pöchhacker, F. (2016). *Introducing interpreting studies* (2nd ed.). London: Routledge.

Roos, C. (2013). Young deaf children's fingerspelling in learning to read and write: An ethnographic study in a signing setting. *Deafness & Education International*, 15(3), 149–178.

Russell, D., Williamson, A., Hayes, J., & Nelson-Julander, A. (2021). Preparation strategies used by interpreters in educational settings: An intervention study. In E. A. Winston & S. B. Fitzmaurice (Eds.), *Advances in educational interpreting* (pp. 147–174). Washington, DC: Gallaudet University Press.

Russell, D., & Winston, B. (2014). Tapping into the interpreting process: Using participant reports to inform the interpreting process in educational settings. *Translation & Interpreting*, 6(1), 102–127.

Schick, B., & Williams, K. (2004). The Educational Interpreter Performance Assessment: Current structure and practices. In E. A. Winston (Ed.), *Educational interpreting: How it can succeed* (pp. 186–205). Washington, DC: Gallaudet University Press.

Schick, B., Williams, K., & Kupermintz, H. (2006). Look who's being left behind: Educational interpreters and access to education for deaf and hard-of-hearing students. *Journal of Deaf Studies and Deaf Education*, 11(1), 3–20.

Schwenke, T. J. (2015). Sign language interpreters and burnout: Exploring perfectionism and coping. *JADARA*, 49(2): 7.

Shaw, S., & Hughes, G. (2006). Essential characteristics of sign language interpreting students: Perspectives of students and faculty. *Interpreting*, 8(2), 195–221.

Stone, A., Kartheiser, G., Hauser, P., Petitto, L., & Allen, T. (2015). Fingerspelling as a novel gateway into reading fluency in deaf bilinguals. *PLoS ONE*, 10(10): e0139610.

Swartz, D. B. (2008). *Burnout among interpreters for the deaf: Implications for educational interpreters* (Master's thesis). Western Oregon University.

Tett, R. P., & Burnett, D. D. (2003). A personality trait-based interactionist model of job performance. *Journal of Applied Psychology*, 88(3), 500–517.

Trezek, B. J., & Malmgren, K. W. (2005). The efficacy of utilizing a phonics treatment package with middle school deaf and hard-of-hearing students. *Journal of Deaf Studies and Deaf Education*, 10(3), 256–271.

Valli, C., Lucas, C., Mulrooney, K. J., & Villanueva, M. (2011). *Linguistics of American Sign Language: An introduction* (5th ed.). Washington, DC: Gallaudet University Press.

Wilcox, S. (1992). *The phonetics of fingerspelling*. Amsterdam: John Benjamins Publishing.

Wilcox, S. (2000). *Metaphor in American Sign Language*. Washington, DC: Gallaudet University Press.

Witter-Merithew, A., & Johnson, L. J. (2005). *Toward competent practice: Conversations with stakeholders*. Alexandria, VA: RID Press.

Yang, C. (2025). Exploring essential personality traits for professional interpreters: A Delphi method study. *Frontiers in Education*, 10: 1597064.

9 Final Thoughts

Educational interpreting is a field of immense complexity, responsibility, and potential impact. It demands more than fluency in languages—it requires cultural competence, pedagogical awareness, critical thinking, and a deep commitment to Deaf students' rights and access. Throughout this text, we have emphasized the cognitive dissonance many interpreters feel: knowing that interpreted education is often far from ideal, yet striving every day to bridge the gaps for students in systems not built for them. This work is challenging because it matters so deeply. It touches lives, shapes identities, and affects educational and personal outcomes. As you move forward in your own practice, let this book serve as a foundation and a call to action: to examine your beliefs, expand your knowledge, connect with diverse Deaf communities, and never stop learning. Educational interpreters are not substitutes—they are specialists. And while the ideal remains direct instruction in fully accessible environments, until that reality exists for all Deaf students, we must bring our best to the work—every day, every class, every child. We close out with our individual perspectives.

Deb

I have spent my entire career as an educational interpreter. I graduated from my Interpreter Program in 2004 and began working for a school district full-time in 2005. I took the Educational Interpreter Performance Assessment (EIPA) in 2007, right around the time the Registry of Interpreters for the Deaf (RID) was debating the now-defunct Ed:K-12 certification. I still remember what RID-certified interpreters said about educational interpreters. I remember searching for workshops about interpreting in educational settings but finding nothing.

When the National Association of Interpreters in Education (NAIE) finally launched in 2016, I cried. That inaugural conference was the very first time in my (at that time, 12-year) career that I had felt seen, validated, and honored as the specialist that I was… for I was, and am, a specialist interpreter in educational interpreting. Believe me when I tell you that this textbook is incredibly personal to me. What I have shared here is born from my 20-plus years of practicing, teaching, mentoring, and researching educational interpreting. I

DOI: 10.4324/9781003423058-9

wrote the textbook that I wanted to have as a new interpreter, and that I want to have as an experienced interpreter and teacher.

I feel compelled to take our own advice and detail some key takeaways I want you to have from this textbook. The first is a heavy irony—educational interpreters should not exist. Not really, and certainly not on the scale at which they do now. When you consider the factors that go into an interpreted education, many Deaf students who have educational interpreter services are not receiving a Free and Appropriate Public Education in their least restrictive environment. They just aren't. They do not have direct access to their teachers and peers. The curriculum, lessons, and pacing are not designed for their linguistic or visual learning needs. This is the point we made at the beginning, and I want to reiterate it now. An interpreted education is not ideal. Period. In some ways, my entire career has been a study in cognitive dissonance. That said, Deaf children do not have time to wait for the system to change. They have right now, and they have the interpreter(s) working with them right now. I hope this text makes you feel at least better prepared for being an educational interpreter in the systems we have today.

Another takeaway is that I want you to examine yourself. *Really* examine yourself. What do you believe about education? About Deaf people? About Deaf communities? About intersectional Deaf identities? What are your privileges (race, sex, gender, expression, orientation, religion, socioeconomic...)? How do your personal, cultural, and professional values inform your decision-making? Why did you decide to get into the interpreting field, and why educational interpreting specifically? Do not answer these questions now. Take them with you and reflect on them often.

Language deprivation is real. It is insidious. Its only cure is prevention. It makes our work exponentially more difficult. When you work with a student who has language deprivation (not if, when), remember that they need context for everything. Don't be afraid to look up images, videos, and to grab a whiteboard and marker. Visual aids help everyone.

Educational interpreting is *hard*. Contrary to what I was told in my interpreter program, implicitly, if not explicitly, educational settings are not a "safe" place for an interpreter to get their on-the-job training. Unfortunately, the perception of educational interpreters by both the education and interpreting fields has resulted in job descriptions, expectations, and pay ranges that are not befitting of a specialist. This textbook is a step in the direction we want to go—to a world where educational interpreting is recognized as an elite specialty in the field of interpreting (if it must exist at all).

Never stop learning. Interpreters need to know stuff about things, and educational interpreters need to know something about everything. This includes popular culture as well as academic subjects. We did not touch on movies, video games, and social media influencers, but these are topics students *will* talk about, including Deaf students. Who knew watching TV and scrolling social media sites would count as prep time? Guess what? It does. Get outside of your echo chamber and learn about what other people play, watch, create—especially if they do not look like you!

Lastly, stay involved with diverse Deaf communities. Do not be that interpreter who never uses ASL outside of work. If the only Deaf person you ever see is the student you are interpreting with, your skills will atrophy, and their language and education will suffer. Make it a habit to seek out the Deaf community, even if it is digitally. Attend workshops in ASL without relying on English interpretation. Challenge yourself to grow.

Stephen

I hope this text has offered you valuable insights and practical tools. For a long time, I've recognized that the resources for teaching educational interpreting have been scattered and insufficiently focused on the unique demands of this field. While there are excellent books discussing research and the current state of educational interpreting—you should definitely seek those out—and while there are solid curricula for teaching general interpreting skills, there's been a clear gap when it comes to addressing the specific nuances of educational interpreting.

Unfortunately, many graduates from interpreting programs enter the field of educational interpreting without an adequate foundation. Novice interpreters working in public schools only worsens the outcomes for Deaf students if their educational interpreters aren't fully prepared for the task. That's why we wrote this book—from both our hearts and extensive experience. I spent a decade working as an educational interpreter, and the past 20 years have been dedicated to supporting in-service educational interpreters. Through this work, I've seen the gaps in foundational knowledge that still exist, and I truly hope this text helps to fill some of those gaps, while also empowering you to explore and build upon the strategies shared here.

I also hope this text will inspire many general interpreting programs across North America to reconsider and revise their curricula. I also believe we need more specialized educational interpreting programs. Educational interpreting is not a lesser version of interpreting for adults—it's fundamentally different. Applying an interpreting-for-adults framework to interpreting for children in educational settings has proven ineffective for over 50 years. I believe this text can serve as a starting point for much-needed curriculum revisions, ensuring that educational interpreters are equipped to meet the unique demands of the job.

As Deb mentioned earlier, educational interpreting is incredibly challenging. Having interpreted in a wide variety of settings—legal, medical, corporate, theological, and more—I can confidently say that no setting is as difficult as interpreting in public schools. But, by the same token, *no setting is as rewarding*.

Seeing a Deaf student's face light up when they finally grasp a concept, watching them confidently answer every math question on a test, or witnessing them raise their hand for the first time to join a class discussion—these moments are beyond rewarding. Even seeing a Deaf student form early friendships with their peers can bring a smile to your face, knowing that your interpreting played a key role in their social and academic development. The work is demanding, but the rewards are priceless.

Of course, we couldn't cover every single aspect that educational interpreters need to know, but I believe we've provided a strong foundation to build upon. At its core, this book has aimed to address how educational interpreters can bridge the gaps for Deaf students by distinguishing between language, modality, and communication. As we've emphasized, language is the bedrock of cognitive and social development, and without early, consistent access to a natural language like ASL, Deaf children face significant challenges both in and out of the classroom.

Despite the progress we've made in recognizing language deprivation, many Deaf students still lack the language foundation they need when they enter school. The ongoing inconsistency in early language exposure and the inadequate support in mainstream education systems continue to hinder their academic and social development. Educational interpreters often find themselves in difficult positions, juggling the need to provide both ASL and English literacy without sufficient training or resources.

To truly close this gap for Deaf students, we need a holistic approach that prioritizes early language acquisition and bilingual education. Educational interpreters must be amazingly skilled and knowledgeable interpreters to ensure Deaf students have the same opportunities for academic success as their hearing peers.

Imagine if every Deaf child entered school with a solid foundation in both ASL and English. A time where educational interpreters, teachers, and families worked together to nurture the cognitive and linguistic growth of Deaf students. Achieving this will require dedication, collaboration, and a deep understanding of the unique needs of Deaf students, but the rewards—an inclusive and equitable educational experience—*will be well worth the effort.*

Experientia nostra te ducat. Egredere et fac bonum opus.

Let our experience guide you. Go forth and do good work.

Glossary

Advanced Placement (AP)	an organization/company that creates curricula that can be taught at the high school level that can provide for students to receive college-level credit if they score at a certain level on the standardized exam.
American College Testing (ACT)	American College Testing, a standardized test used for college admissions in the United States.
Boys Town National Research Hospital (BTNRH)	a non-profit research and medical center in Nebraska serving as the home for the Educational Interpreter Performance Assessment Diagnostic Center.
Classifier	a specific handshape used in American Sign Language (ASL) to represent a category or "class" of nouns and to convey detailed visual information about those nouns—such as their size, shape, movement, location, or how they interact with other objects. Classifiers are not standalone signs but rather part of a grammatical system in ASL that enhances spatial and descriptive meaning. Modern research refers to classifiers as depiction.
Code of Professional Conduct (CPC)	the interpreter's Code of Professional Conduct promulgated by the Registry of Interpreters for the Deaf (RID) as ethical tenets to guide professional interpreters in the United States.
Compressions	the ways in which information is condensed in American Sign Language (ASL) compared to spoken English. If the amount of detail in the source language is too great, an interpreter must compress the information in the target language.

Conceptually Accurate Signed English (CASE)	a communication method drawing some signs from American Sign Language (ASL) while attempting to use the basic grammar and rules of English.
Cued Language	a visual communication system using cues or handshapes and locations to convey phonemes. Sometimes called Cued Speech, this system is not used widely.
Deaf Education (DeafEd)	education which typically involves Deaf students with an Individualized Education Program (IEP) and uses Teachers of the Deaf (ToD) to teach Deaf students.
Demand-Control Schema (DCS)	a schema adapted by Dean and Pollard as a structure for interpreters to use when making decisions based on environmental, interpersonal, paralinguistic, and intrapersonal demands.
Educational Interpreter Code of Ethics (EICOE)	a set of professional guidelines designed specifically for interpreters working in K–12 educational settings. Written by the National Association of Interpreters in Education (NAIE), it establishes standards of conduct to protect the rights, confidentiality, and dignity of Deaf students while ensuring effective and appropriate communication access in the classroom.
Educational Interpreter Performance Assessment (EIPA)	a psychometrically valid examination to determine the skills of an educational interpreter using a comprehensive rating system. The EIPA is widely used in the United States and Canada.
Educational Interpreter Performance Assessment Written Test (EIPA:WT)	a widely used evaluation of an interpreter's knowledge competencies needed to work with students in an educational setting. The EIPA:WT is widely used in the United States and Canada.
Educational K-12 (Ed:K-12) Certification	a national certification issued by the Registry of Interpreters for the Deaf (RID) to interpreter members who scored an EIPA 4.0 or higher, passed the EIPA:WT, and held a baccalaureate degree. This certification was discontinued in 2016.
Emergency Operations Plan (EOP)	a comprehensive, formal document that outlines how a school will respond to various types of emergencies or disasters. The goal of an EOP is to ensure the safety of individuals, minimize damage, and restore normal operations as quickly as possible.

Expansions	ways in which information is expanded in American Sign Language (ASL) compared to spoken English. If the amount of detail in the source language is insufficient in the target language an interpreter must expand the information.
Extralinguistic Knowledge (ELK)	any knowledge an interpreter may possess outside of the topic or information being presented.
Federal Department of Education (FDE)	the United States Department of Education (FDE) is a federal department responsible for establishing policies, administering and coordinating federal assistance to education, collecting data, and enforcing federal educational laws regarding privacy and civil rights.
FM/DM	a frequency modulation/digital modulation system that transmits sound through either radio waves or digital signals. These systems are sometimes used by Deaf students in classrooms.
Graphic Organizer	a visual learning tool that helps students organize their ideas.
Information Processing: Bottom-up	is when you think about the words in a discourse. An example of this would be thinking, "How do I sign 'mitosis, anaphase, prophase, telophase…'?" rather than focusing on the fact that mitosis is a process with five phases.
Information Processing: Top-down	is when the goal and main ideas of a discourse drive your interpretation. Top-down processing includes summaries and outlines.
Interpreter	a trained professional who works between languages by co-constructing the source language in the target language ensuring that the meaning, intent, and tone of the original message are accurately preserved. An interpreter works after a one-time exposure in real time (or near real time) so that the interpretation is typically only accessible at that time.
Local Education Agency (LEA)	a United States federal term for a public authority responsible for the administration of public education within a specific geographic area. Typically, LEAs are referred to as a school district or precinct.
Morpheme	the smallest unit of meaning in a language. Morphemes cannot be broken down into smaller parts that carry meaning. There are free morphemes which can stand alone as words (e.g., book, cat, happy). There are also bound morphemes which

	must be attached to another morpheme to convey meaning. For example, in English, -s in books conveying plural, un- in unhappy to convey negation, or -ing in walking to convey present progressive form. In American Sign Language (ASL), free morphemes include the signs MOTHER, EAT, BLUE. Bound morphemes among others may include movement changes to show tense, number, or aspect, or non-manual signals or expressions that change the meaning.
Morphology	the structure and formation of words or signs. It focuses on morphemes, which are the smallest units of meaning in a language.
Multidisciplinary Team (MDT)	in an educational context, a group of professionals that conducts assessments to determine if a student qualifies for special education services. This may include psychologists, medical doctors, social workers, speech language pathologists, teachers, and others.
National Association of Interpreters in Education (NAIE)	an American non-profit organization that promotes best practices and professional standards for educational interpreters working with Deaf students.
Omissions	instances where the interpreter leaves out information that was present in the source message. Omissions can be intentional or unintentional and due to processing limitations, lack of understanding, fatigue, time constraints, or decisions made to improve clarity or relevance. While some omissions may be strategic and ethically justifiable, frequent or critical omissions can impact the accuracy and completeness of the interpreted message, potentially affecting communication access.
Phonology	branch of linguistics concerned with the systematic organization of sounds in languages. It studies how sounds function within a particular language or languages, including the rules for combining them, how they interact, and how they are perceived and produced. In signed languages like American Sign Language (ASL), phonology refers to the organization of features such as handshape, movement, location, palm orientation, and facial expressions.

Physical Education (PE)	a planned curriculum to develop motor skills, knowledge, and behaviors for active living and physical fitness. Sometimes colloquially referred to as Gym Class.
Pidgin Signed English (PSE)	a dated and incorrect term for Contact Sign that blends elements of American Sign Language (ASL) and English. PSE is not a standardized language and typically follows English word order more closely than ASL but uses ASL vocabulary and some grammatical features.
Positive Behavioral Interventions and Supports (PBIS)	an evidence-based framework used in schools to improve student behavior and create positive learning environments. PBIS focuses on teaching and reinforcing appropriate behaviors, preventing challenging behaviors, and using data to guide decision-making. It operates on a tiered model of support for behavioral, academic, social, emotional, and mental health offering increasing levels of intervention based on student needs.
Registry of Interpreters for the Deaf (RID)	a national certifying body for community-based sign language interpreters. RID serves as a professional membership organization that seeks to uphold standards, ethics, and professionalism for interpreters working with Deaf communities.
Sapir–Whorf Hypothesis	a theory that states language determines or influences a person's thought. People using different languages may see the world differently based on how they use language to describe it.
Scholastic Assessment Test (SAT)	a standardized college admissions test in the United States that measures a high school student's readiness for college. The SAT assesses skills in reading, writing, and mathematics and is used by college admissions processes.
Seeing Essential English (SEE I)	a manually coded English system developed in the 1960s that represents English visually by using signs for every English word and grammatical marker, including articles, plurals, and verb endings. It uses invented signs to represent English morphemes in strict word order to reinforce English grammar and syntax, often resulting in unnatural signing for native American Sign Language (ASL) users.
Sequential Affixation	attaching an affix (prefix or suffix) to a base word.

Signing Exact English (SEE II)	a 1972 invented, updated version of SEE I which also aims to represent English visually through signs, maintaining English word order and grammar. It includes fewer invented signs than SEE I and attempts to use American Sign Language (ASL) signs where possible while adding affixes and word endings. SEE II is more commonly used than SEE I but is still a manually coded system, not a natural language, and is not widely used among Deaf communities.
Simultaneous Communication (SimCom)	a communication method used by some Deaf individuals that combines both sign language and spoken language simultaneously. In SimCom, a person signs while speaking (or vice versa) and it is often used in situations where communication needs to be accessible to both Deaf and hearing individuals. Research indicates this approach is ineffective at conveying both languages and codes but may be somewhat useful for hard-of-hearing students.
Special Education (SPED)	a specialized form of education designed to meet the unique needs of students with disabilities. It involves individualized instruction and support to help students with physical, emotional, behavioral, or learning challenges to succeed in school. Special education services may include adaptations to the curriculum, teaching methods, classroom environment, and the use of specialized equipment or technology. Special education is governed by laws such as the Individuals with Disabilities Education Act (IDEA), which ensures that students with disabilities receive a free and appropriate public education (FAPE).
Speech Language Pathologist (SLP)	a professional who diagnoses and treats speech, language, and communication disorders. In educational settings, SLPs work with students who have speech or language delays, including Deaf students, to improve their communication skills. They often collaborate with teachers, parents, and other professionals to support students' learning and development.
State Department of Education (SDE)	a United States federal term to represent the state-level agency responsible for overseeing public education.

Teacher of the Deaf (ToD)	a certified teaching professional with a background in Deaf education and who works with students who are Deaf or hard of hearing. A ToD's role includes developing Individualized Education Programs (IEPs); providing direct instruction in subjects such as reading, writing, math, and social studies; and collaborating with other professionals.
Translator	a person who works with written language by co-constructing the source language in the target language. Unlike interpreters, who work with spoken or signed language in real time, translators focus solely on static language materials (such as print or video) and have continuous exposure to the source language.
Transliterator	a person who works between a spoken language such as English and Contact Sign, Manually Coded English (MCE), or another such sign coding system.
Visual Phonics	an instructional tool of 45 hand gestures and symbols that represent the phonemes of spoken English. While aimed at providing some visual cue to phonetic awareness, it has limited practical application and no broad empirical evidence this strategy works.
Vocational Rehabilitation Act (Section 504)	a United States federal civil rights law that prohibits discrimination against individuals with disabilities in programs and activities that receive federal financial assistance, including public schools. Under Section 504, eligible students with physical or mental impairments that substantially limit one or more major life activities are entitled to receive accommodations and modifications to ensure equal access to education.

Index

Note: Locators in *italic* and **bold** refer figures and tables respectively

Printed in the United States
by Baker & Taylor Publisher Services